MW01245436

This Book Includes 2 Parts:

Mediterranean Diet For Beginners AND Fat Loss For Women And Men

By Laura Violet & James Moore

Table of Contents

PARTI I - Mediterranean Diet
For Beginners

Introduction

Everyone has their own take on the ideal meal. In most cases though, it consists of high fat, high salt and high sugar foods. Indeed this has been the notion of home cooking made by good old mom.

Who is not used to the smell of bacon and pancakes at the breakfast table anyway? Come dinner time, a huge slab of red meat with a side of mashed potatoes and buttered vegetables is ripe for the picking. This is how most people would picture the perfect meal.

The result is that this kind of eating habit and diet has gone down as a lifestyle. It takes root from the post-war victory that the Western World enjoyed and became one of the most visible evidence of their prosperity.

Current Obesity Trends

Based on the staggering figures from WHO, approximately 2/3rds of all Americans adults can be classed as overweight. All of the high calorie hamburgers, sundaes, French fries, sodas, cheese cakes, ice cream and other popular food items are taking its toll. Even though American maintains the lead, as in many other areas, they are not alone in this problem because many other countries are now following the same patterns. If these current trends are not halted, the prediction for 2030 is nearly half of all Americans may be obese. While this problem is big and massive to the world, the change that occurs can be drilled down to a one-on-one choice. This means, if no one makes a change, it is up to the individual to take the information that they have learned and act on it.

Sadly, the same eating habits have made America and other parts of the Western World a haven for heart attack and other heart disease-related deaths per year. Nowadays, most people struggle to regain their health and live a healthier lifestyle.

This sudden health consciousness has prompted scientists and nutritionist to look for healthier eating habits.

Over the years, they began to realize that the future of nutritious diets is actually in traditional cuisine. In the 1950s and 1960s, researchers noted of the relatively low budget but healthier diets enjoyed by people in the Mediterranean region.

While America and the rest of the Western World celebrated their post-war victory and prosperity, the Mediterranean region continued living the way they have been for centuries.

This is actually the very reason for the low number of cases of coronary heart disease and other such conditions. Researchers were stunned to find that plant-based diets are actually better than animal-based diets.

As the evidence points out, the Mediterranean diet is definitely a healthier way to eat. This diet is actually based on the diet of a region and not just once country.

The Mediterranean is the world's largest inland sea which borders Europe, Africa and Asia. Around fifteen countries including France, Spain, Greece, Portugal and Italy among others call this region home.

The Mediterranean diet and way of life may take root from various countries but they do follow a similar pattern. All in all, this diet consists of whole grain, legumes, dried beans and a wide range of fruits and vegetables. Red meats are taken in small amounts and in some cases not at all.

It is this kind of diet that has helped people from this part of the world to stay healthy.

A healthier body and lifestyle is certainly within your grasp thanks to the Mediterranean diet. This eBook is meant to be your personal guide to exploring this healthy diet. It also teaches you valuable tips on improving your health.

You will soon learn of all the benefits of this diet in the long term. For your convenience, a few recipes and meal plans are included as well. Say goodbye to your old unhealthy diet and be ready to set sail towards a healthier you.

Chapter One: What is Mediterranean Diet

The Mediterranean is one of the world's premier tourist destinations. A lot of people dream of spending their vacation here some day. Its beauty and charm mostly comes from its rich history and culture.

The warm feeling of the sun on the skin and the calm sea breeze are things to look forward to as well. Yet these are not the only reasons for crowds of people flocking to this part of the world.

Apart from being exceptionally unique in taste, the Mediterranean cuisine has proven to be one of the worlds healthiest. Years' worth of research has helped shed light on the mysteries of this diet.

Specifically, how delicious and savory food can be good for the health at the same time. This healthy cuisine comes from a mixture of European, Asian and North African origin which produces truly unique dishes.

The Lay of the Land

The reason behind the Mediterranean diet's diversity lies in its geography itself. All territories around the Mediterranean Sea are the origins of this diet. This region stretches from the Straits of Gibraltar all the way across the shores of the Middle East.

Parts of Southern Spain and the seaport of Tangier in

Northern Morocco are included as well. This vast tract of territory plays host to some of the world's richest and diverse cultures.

The wide range of countries and cultures each has its unique contribution to the Mediterranean diet. Even with the distinct flavors of each culture, the diet has retained a few common characteristics.

Pasta may be known as ziti in Italy but the same variant exists in Morocco as couscous. Apart from food, Mediterranean people share a distinct attitude towards food and the manner it is eaten. This is the result of centuries of interactions which continues to evolve to this day.

Eating à la Mediterranean

Taking part in the traditional Mediterranean diet is mostly a seasonal and regional thing. In general, each country produces foods locally and is served soon after harvest with each country having its own customs.

Fresh vegetables harvested in the spring and are eaten usually within a few miles from the farm. The same thing happens during the summer with lots of tomatoes, cantaloupes, eggplants and watermelons among others.

When summer ends, wine pressing begins with harvests of olives following suit. Later on, you will learn how all these come together in the Mediterranean diet.

As such, outdoor markets are full of ripe and vibrantly-colored fruits and vegetables fresh from the farm. This is certainly not the same as the pale and bland produce you are used to from the supermarket.

Now who would want to eat that after sampling some Mediterranean produce?

Red meat is simply lacking in Mediterranean cuisine due to the lack of grazing land. In its place, lamb and veal are served although sparingly and only for special occasions. You are more likely to encounter chicken or seafood in main courses.

Bread is a staple in this diet especially in Italy where it is consumed readily. This bread is dark, heavy and packed with whole grains unlike the one from the supermarket though.

Pasta and rice are famous as well. Legumes are a good source of protein and are more affordable than meat. Lentils, chickpeas, small red cranberry beans and fava beans remain popular choices today.

Of course you cannot talk about Mediterranean cuisine without talking about wine. The difference here is that this is consumed with meals and never for recreation.

Eating cheese is a common way to start and end a meal but never in the same way as Americanized Italian dishes.

The similar flavor shared by a lot of Mediterranean dishes is thanks in part to the flavorings used. More often than not, this includes onion, garlic, lemons, basil, oregano and of course olive oil.

Beyond the food itself, Mediterranean cuisine sets itself apart because of the way it sees food. It is a philosophy which regards food and eating as a way sustain the vitality of life.

It is a means by which life can be expressed in all its beauty.

Friends and family gather around and eat together in genuine events and not inconvenient chores. In other words, food is a reflection of one's life.

Discovering the Diet

Beginning in the 1950s, the Mediterranean diet has received increasing attention over the years. Keep in mind that this was the time when Americans much on steak dinners and baked potatoes with a side of buttered bread rolls and a glass of whole milk. This was thought to be the ideal nutritious diet of the day. Numerous studies have been conducted and all with the same astonishing conclusions.

Research has revealed that people taking the Mediterranean diet have a lesser tendency to develop cardiovascular diseases and cancer. This is due to the homemade meals which use fresh ingredients and low servings of red meat. Because of this and the Mediterranean way of life, people from this region tend to live longer as well.

Among the most well-known studies into the Mediterranean diet is the Seven Countries Study by Ancel Keys in the 1950s and 1960s. This included a sample population from Greece, Italy, the former Yugoslavia, Finland, the Netherlands, Japan and the United States.

Specifically, the study explored the relationship between disease and diet. It involved over 12,000 men between the ages of 40 and 59. The study revealed that men taking the Mediterranean diet were less likely to contract coronary heart disease.

Later studies proved that a diet low in saturated fat reduces cholesterol levels and the risk of heart disease. The Mediterranean diet mainly consists of monounsaturated fat which is the good kind of fat that your body needs. This good fat is mainly from olive oil which is a mainstay in most Mediterranean dishes.

Research still continues to have a better understanding into the links between lower risk of heart disease and the Mediterranean diet. Apart from the diet, research now points towards increased activity as part of the lifestyle as another cause for this figure.

The lifestyle in the Mediterranean is more relaxed with strong support from friends and family.

Compare DASH and Mediterranean diet

Both the DASH (Dietary Approaches to Stop Hypertension) and the Mediterranean diet plan are healthy nutritional plans for your body. The DASH diet was developed as a flexible eating plan to reduce hypertension by the National heart, Lung and Blood institute.

The dietary plan was studied with the goal of reducing high blood pressure. The diet is low in saturated fats, cholesterol, total fat, and sweets. It is high in fruit, vegetables, fat-free or low-fat dairy products, whole grains, fish, poultry, beans, seeds and nuts.

This plan is also lower in salt content that the standard Western diet. According to the Mayo Clinic the standard Western diet delivers approximately 3500 mg of salt per day, while the DASH diet recommends no more than 2300 and will recommend 1500 to patients who already have high blood pressure.

Proponents of the diet do not advocate using salt substitutes that can be higher in chemical potassium not found naturally in foods and can be more harmful to individuals who already have cardiovascular or kidney problems. Instead, they recommend reducing your sodium intake and substituting other herbs and spices that are sodium free but which add flavor to your foods.

The Mediterranean diet also has significant health benefits. Researchers have found that it reduces your risk of diabetes and can significantly level your blood sugar among other benefits.

The diet describes a specific mix of foods that developed across 16 different countries which border the Mediterranean sea. However, while there is a variety of cooking styles and foods, there are several consistent factors which appear to be the basis for the identified health benefits. There is not a strict list of foods that you can and cannot eat, nor is there one or two superfoods that must be included.

Instead, the underlying basic principles of the diet include foods that are high in vegetables, peas and beans. The amount of red meat is limited and people eat more poultry and fish. Although the diet is high in fats, the fat is monounsaturated fat, like that found in olive oil and grapeseed oil. Animal fat is limited, as is processed fast foods and those high in trans fats.

The diet is high in water, limits sodas and other drinks but does advocate one or two small glasses of red wine with dinner. No salt is added at the table and very minimal is added during cooking.

The largest difference between the two diets is the amount and types of fat that are recommended. The Mediterranean diet is high in fats from nuts, seeds and added olive oils to foods while the DASH diet recommends a lower fat version of products.

Although each does have health benefits, the Mediterranean diet also will help to reduce blood pressure measurement and reduce cardiovascular risk while also ensuring the necessary fat content for optimal brain health

Chapter Two: Fats

What are MUFAs

The term MUFA is an acronym that stands for MonoUnsaturated Fatty Acids and is pronounced moo-fah. These fatty acids are plant based and are often found in some delicious foods like avocados, olive oils, nuts, seeds, olives and dark chocolate.

MUFAs are an integral part of the Mediterranean diet, popular in over 16 countries found around the Mediterranean sea. While each of these countries eat a diet that has variety, they also do have some consistent characteristics, which include the use of MUFA foods.

These foods, while healthy, are also high in fat. Foods that are high in fat are also higher in calories than other foods. While foods that are higher in fats are more calorie dense, they also keep you feeling full longer and can mean you eat less foods. In fact, people who consistently eat a Mediterranean style diet plan are less likely to be overweight or obese.

Other benefits to eating a diet high in monounsaturated fatty acids include a reduced risk of breast cancer, lower cholesterol levels and a lower risk of heart disease and stroke. People who have rheumatoid arthritis may also experience less severe pain and stiffness.

MUFAs are healthy fats, and by replacing saturated fats, trans fats, and any other unhealthy fats with the healthy variants of unsaturated fats like MUFA and polyunsaturated fats, you will be able to improve your heart's health. MUFAs help reduce the levels of LDL (low-density lipoprotein) while increasing the share of HDL (high-density lipoprotein). Do these terms seem too technical? Well, these lipoproteins are what cholesterol is made of. Did you know that not all types of cholesterol are harmful? Yes, you read that right! HDL is believed to be the "good" cholesterol, whereas LDL is the undesirable one. By increasing the levels of HDL, your heart's health will automatically improve and this, in turn, will reduce the risk of any potential heart diseases. Also, MUFAs can help in improving the function of the blood vessels within your body. It can also help in controlling the levels of insulin as well as blood sugar. When these two levels don't fluctuate, it helps in preventing and managing diabetes.

MUFAs are quite an important part of the Mediterranean diet. There are various foods that are high in MUFAs like olive oil, canola oil, avocados, almonds, pecans, cashews, macadamias, different nut butters, olives, and peanut oil, and they are all an integral part of the Mediterranean diet.

Research published in the Archives of Internal Medicine found that individuals who ate a diet high in MUFAs may have a protective effect on the risk of breast cancer. Research published in the American journal of clinical Nutrition found that diets that were high in monounsaturated fatty acids lowered both total cholesterol and triglyceride concentrations; however, one of the benefits to eating a diet high in MUFAs that is very popular is a reduction in belly fat. In a study published by the American Diabetes Association, researchers found that a diet that was rich in MUFAs would prevent the deposition of central fat, or belly fat. They also found that it reduces insulin resistance and improves insulin sensitivity.

What Is Omega 3 & Why Is It Healthy?

Considered one of the essential fatty acids, Omega 3s are essential to human health.

The problem is our bodies are unable to make them on their own! So that leaves the food we eat as our main source of Omega 3.

Of course, we can, and most of us should, also take an Omega 3 supplement to ensure that our body has all of the important fatty acids that it needs to build muscles and maintain proper cell growth.

Omega 3s are considered a polyunsaturated fatty acid (PUFA) that is crucial to maintain proper brain function, growth and development.

An important anti-inflammatory, one of Omega 3's jobs is to help prevent such degenerative diseases as arthritis, cancer, heart disease, and even memory loss.

Of course, Omega 3s also aid in keeping skin taut and smooth, thus playing an important role in keeping us looking younger longer. From warding off wrinkles, to helping to keep coronary arteries clear, Omega 3 fatty acids have been linked to all sorts of health benefits, which we will discuss in detail in the upcoming pages.

Let's look at the three main types of Omega 3 fatty acids: EPA, DHA and ALA.

Eicosapentaenoic Acid (EPA)

EPA is a very important Omega 3 fatty acid. New research indicates that EPA can actually prevent a heart attack or stroke. One study even reported that people with low levels of EPA in their body are as much as 47% more likely to suffer a cardiac episode than those with sufficient levels of EPA in their system.

To keep a sufficient amount of EPA in your system, you would need to eat between 400 and 500 grams of cold water fish such as sardines, mackerel, or salmon 2-3 times per week. Few people, unfortunately, can stomach that much deep-sea fish.

Even if you could, most experts warn against it since so many of the world's fish are now contaminated with mercury and other toxins.

So what's the alternative? Taking 1,000 mg of EPA rich fish oil on a daily basis is considered by most experts to work well at keeping EPA blood levels just as high as eating large amounts of deep sea fish. Keep in mind though, that EPA also needs DHA in order to work properly, so be sure any supplement you buy contains both.

What Is DHA?

Docosahexaenoic Acid (DHA) is another very important Omega 3 fatty acid needed by the body to achieve optimal health. It is one of the longest chains of PUFAs found in Omega 3s. It is also essential to good brain function. Nearly one fourth of the brain is made up of DHA and without this important fat, you can suffer from several mental disorders, depression, or even Attention Deficit Disorder (ADD)!

In fact, scientific research has demonstrated a correlation between increased DHA levels and decreased incidence of Alzheimer's Disease. Worse yet, without the right amount of DHA, your brain is unable to tell all of your organs what to do. Your heart can't beat and your lungs can't breathe without an order from your brain.

Even if a low DHA level doesn't cause your body to go into catastrophic breakdown, it can leave you susceptible to a myriad of diseases or illness.

Now that you know how important getting the right amount of DHA is to overall health and wellbeing, you may be wondering what your best source of it is... fish oil.

You can get DHA laden fish oil in one of two ways:

By eating more fatty fish or by taking a DHA supplement. Either way, the important thing to remember is that both EPA and DHA are crucial Omega 3 fatty acids that you must get regularly in order to ward off disease.

Why is ALA Fatty Acids So Important?

Found mainly in dark green, leafy vegetables, flax seed, and walnuts, Alpha-Linolenic Acid (ALA) can do something other Omega 3 fatty acids can't: if your body needs them, it can convert ALA into both DHA and EPA. This is a unique and wonderful ability, since our bodies needs these important Omega 3 fatty acids to stay healthy.

Omega 3 fatty acids are the good fats in our healthy diets. They are the fats our body needs to properly function.

They help keep our heart functioning at a healthy rate. Keeps our brains functioning as we age and help infants gain information.

Omega acids also help keep our joints functioning.

While our diet recommends we limit our oil and fat consumption, we do need them. Fat and oil help keep our bodies at our peak

performance. Fat is what keeps our bodies on the move, this is why it is best to get the healthier versions. The healthy oils provided by fatty acids help keep the fats consumed from turning into heart clogging cholesterol. This is also avoided when you limit your fat intake in your diet.

While adding Omega 3 fatty acids to your diet does have health benefits always discuss with your doctor. They will be able to provide resources for what source works best for your diet.

We have all heard the speech given that we need a healthy diet. Over the decades this became an issue with the invention of snack foods. It became easier to just grab the unhealthy snack foods instead of finding healthier alternatives. This is why the average diet is full of unhealthy fat, salt, and sugar.

Over the decades, we have seen the health problems involved with this diet. Including diabetes, heart attacks, cholesterol issues, hypertension of the heart, obesity. When you are used to an unhealthy diet it gets harder to reverse it properly. This process is much less complicated if you start with small changes and keep them so they become habits. This process can take up to a month of doing the new changes for it to become a habit.

Where Do They Come From?

While the Omega 3 and 6 acids are essential to our bodies, we do not produce them on our own. We can only get these acids by food or supplement sources. Our bodies absorb the natural sources much easier.

This is why doctors recommend to adopt a Mediterranean diet, eating fish and nuts for those deficient in fatty acids. You want your diet to be varied in the sources in which you get these acids. This helps to prevent you becoming bored with the foods you are eating. You can do this by eating a large variety of the fish available as well as the nuts, seeds, and plants.

DHA and EPA are found in fish such as halibut, salmon, anchovies, blue fish, mackerel, trout, bass, sardines and tuna. Keep in mind wild salmon fish has more omega 3 acids than the farmed variety. It is the same with the trout, the lake trout have more acids than the farmed trout. You can get fish from your local butcher, fishmonger, or grocery stores.

While it is more expensive in some areas the health benefits outweigh the costs. If possible find sales, or even go fishing this will reduce costs. Fish can be frozen for later consumption just make sure to check for pin bones to reduce the risk of choking. It is also recommended that pregnant women not eat farmed fish or blue tuna. They both have a higher risk of contaminants such as mercury, lead, and pesticides.

ALA Is found in walnuts, flax seeds and oil canola oil, soybeans and soybean oils. Smaller amounts of the acids are found in dark leafy greens such as kale, spinach and some varieties of lettuce. It is also found in sunflower seeds and oil, cashews, pumpkin seeds and peanuts. This is why doctors recommend things like mixed nuts to help obtain this fatty acid. Dark leafy greens are also a source of iron essential for hemoglobin production in the blood.

Note: It is recommended that young children do not eat nuts until they are four years old at the minimum

Well that's a basic introduction into what Omega 3 is and why it is so healthy.

Chapter Three: Mediterranean Diet Myths

Please don't be under any misconceptions that you can get away with eating extremely fatty foods in large quantities, plenty of carbs and cheese, and expect the scale to take a nosedive. Unless you include some form of exercise or physical activity into your daily schedule, your body will not be able to burn all the calories you consume. One of the reasons the people living in the Mediterranean region are fit is because of a healthy diet that's combined with plenty of physical labor. So, if you truly want to optimize the benefits of this diet, I suggest that you include some sort of exercise along with the diet.

The Mediterranean diet isn't a vegetarian or a vegan diet. A traditional Mediterranean diet does concentrate a lot on plant-based foods, but it isn't merely restricted to those. It is a popular misconception that this diet solely consists of plant-based foods, which could not be further from the truth. The Mediterranean diet is a healthy mixture of plant and animal-based foods that help in optimizing your overall fitness. This diet isn't merely about the food you eat, but is a way of life. It is all about slowing down and enjoying food - and life. It is about practicing mindfulness while eating.

When something is popular, all the curiosity about it usually gives rise to different myths. These myths are the result of misinterpreted information, misconceptions, and uninformed opinions. In this section, you will learn about popular myths and the corresponding facts about the

Mediterranean diet.

Restricted only to the Mediterranean

Just because it is named the Mediterranean diet, that doesn't mean that it cannot work anywhere outside the Mediterranean region. The diet is named so because of the region it originated from. This diet is a way of eating and as with any other way of eating, it can be used by anyone living anywhere in the world. There might be some foods that are specific to this region, but it will do you some good to keep in mind that the Mediterranean region is quite vast and includes a variety of foods. Also, the types of foods included in a typical Mediterranean diet can be procured from anywhere. For instance, there are certain foods that are specific to the North American region, like blueberries, but they can be easily included in the Mediterranean diet, too. So, please don't be under any misconception that the foods included in the Mediterranean diet aren't available anywhere outside the Mediterranean region.

It is all about cheese, pasta and pizza

Yes, these foods are a part of the Mediterranean diet, but that's not what the Mediterranean diet is all about. There are multiple countries as well as cultures in the Mediterranean region, and this diet includes all these variations. The countries present along the coast of the Mediterranean Sea include southern regions of Italy, France, Spain, and Greece along with Turkey, Morocco,

Lebanon, and several other regions. Please keep in mind that the Mediterranean diet is merely a plant-based diet that concentrates on the inclusion of freshly available produce, lots of fish, limited quantities of red meats, and barely any processed foods. So, keeping these basic criteria in mind, it is unfair to say that the Mediterranean diet is merely restricted to cheese, pizza, and pasta.

It is high in fat

The different types of fats that are included within the Mediterranean diet are good for improving your heart health and aren't the ones that promote cholesterol or weight gain. In fact, all the research shows the opposite of the myth. The Mediterranean diet constitutes high amounts of Omega-3 fatty acids and nutritious nuts that help in improving one's overall health. Fat isn't always unhealthy, and by including the right fats in your daily diet, you will be able to improve your fitness and health. It isn't about the amount of fat that's included in your meals, but the type of fat used which makes all the difference. As mentioned earlier, nuts, olive oil, and fish (the main constituents of the Mediterranean diet) contain polyunsaturated and monounsaturated fats. These fats help in improving the heart's health. A typical Mediterranean style of eating contains relatively low levels of saturated fats and most of the saturated fat that are present come in the form of small quantities of cheese or yogurt. So, these fats aren't all that unhealthy, especially when the ingredients they are present in happen to be fermented. Fermented products like yogurt are high in probiotics that help in improving the gut's health. I suggest that it is time to let go of the fat-phobia and start including foods that are naturally healthy to your diet.

You cannot cook with olive oil

The Mediterranean diet includes different types of olive oils. In fact, you are free to choose the type of olive oil you are willing to cook with - virgin olive oil, extra virgin olive oil or pure olive oil. Olive oil will lend your food a rather unique flavor, but it certainly is safe to cook with. Yes, the smoking point of olive oils is relatively lower than that of the other oils used for cooking like vegetable oil or canola oil. However, the smoke point of olive oil is high enough that it can be used for all types of cooking.

In fact, olive oil is used for cooking in almost all of the Mediterranean countries, especially Greece. The smoke point of the olive oil is also dependent on its quality, age, and the condition it is in. Olive oil of good quality can be cooked safely anywhere between the temperatures of 340-410°F. Good quality olive oil is usually enriched with antioxidants, and they help protect the oil from burning. However, if the oil is not of good quality or if it has gone rancid, then the smoke point will be quite low. How can you tell whether the olive oil that you are using is of good quality or not? There is a simple test that you can do - take a spoonful of olive oil and swallow it up. If you feel a slight burn at the back of your throat, then the polyphenols are present in the oil and it means that the oil is good. Polyphenols belong to the group of phytonutrients that contain antioxidant properties.

It is hard to follow

The Mediterranean diet isn't difficult and it is as easy as following a healthy and nutritious plan of eating. If you are trying to focus on increasing the consumption of certain food groups while cutting down on the consumption of others, then it might be a little challenging initially. However, after a while, you will get used to it and it will become rather easy to follow. Following any new diet is similar to adopting a new habit - it takes a while and it requires some patience.

So, why is it important to understand the popular myths about this diet? This is important so that you can make an informed decision. As you become aware of the different benefits that the Mediterranean diet offers, it will not be fair to judge it based on certain misconceptions.

Is the Mediterranean Ideal for you?

How can you possibly decide whether a specific diet is ideal for you or not? Here are a couple of things that you should keep in mind while considering the Mediterranean diet.

The Mediterranean diet is not restrictive and is easy to follow. It obviously isn't possible to follow a diet that isn't practical, and this diet is more than doable. In fact, it is sustainable in the long run too, and anyone can follow it. There are variations of flavors and ingredients for you to choose from. So, you can rest easy knowing that you will never run out of options. Also, the different recipes provided in this book will help you cook tasty and nutritious food that you will never tire of. Another good thing about this diet is that it doesn't require the elimination of any food group. Instead of excluding a food group, you merely make it a point to limit the intake of carbs, sugars and processed foods. By doing all of this, you will automatically be eating healthier than you were before.

The wide variety of produce makes it easy to cook while following this diet. You can still eat the foods you like, provided you tweak them a little. For instance, if you love pizza, you merely need to make sure that the pizza base you use is whole-grain or gluten-free and includes plenty of veggies. Also, topping it with crumbled feta cheese instead of layers of processed cheese makes it healthier than a regular cheese pizza. You can fill yourself up with nutritious food that will keep you feeling fuller for longer and you don't have to worry about starving yourself.

When you are following this diet, your hunger pangs will reduce. This is primarily due to the healthy fats and the fibrous foods included in the meals. By cutting down on red meats and replacing the unhealthy oils with monounsaturated fats in the form of fatty fish, avocados, olive oil and lots of nuts, you will feel quite full for longer. These fats also help in decreasing your cholesterol levels while reducing the potential of any heart diseases. The Mediterranean diet will help reduce the risk of several heart diseases while improving your cognition. Apart from this, it is also a great way to tackle and manage type-2 diabetes.

However, this diet does restrict the intake of milk. So, it means that your calcium levels can deplete if you aren't cautious. Don't you worry, because this can be easily fixed! You merely need to increase your intake of vegetables that are rich in calcium. If you want, you can always take a calcium supplement. Also, please keep in mind that milk isn't the only source of calcium, and the different dairy products prescribed by this diet will ensure that your bones stay healthy while your body gets all the calcium it needs.

Additionally, if you enjoy having a drink every now and then, unlike with other diets, you don't have to give up on alcohol while following the Mediterranean diet. The only catch is that red wine is the only alcohol you can consume that is "approved" by the Mediterranean diet guidelines. An occasional glass of red wine every now and then is good for you and is good for your heart's health, too. The one thing that you must be mindful of is the quantity of fats that you consume. The Mediterranean diet encourages the consumption of naturally fatty foods but is careful about the portions you consume.

If all of this sounds good to you, then following this diet will be quite easy!

Compatibility with Other Diets

The Mediterranean diet is a simple dieting protocol and it is versatile enough to be combined with other diets. If you want to speed up the process of weight loss and are looking to magnify the health benefits this diet offers, I suggest that you combine it with other diets. In this section, you will learn about two different dieting protocols that you can easily combine with the Mediterranean diet.

Keto diet

The Mediterranean diet is quite interesting in terms of all the options it provides. Its practicability combined with the different health benefits it offers make it a nice diet to follow. If you are interested in speeding up the process of weight loss, however, then you should combine it with the ketogenic diet.

During the '80s, the entire western world was gripped by the fear of fats. Fats were demonized, and all sorts of "low-fat" products started cropping up. When you start consuming fewer fats, you automatically start relying heavily on carbs for satiating your hunger. This is one of the reasons behind problems like obesity and diabetes becoming an epidemic. Fat-phobia did more harm than good. However, this perception is slowly changing.

All the carbs that you ingest are broken down into simple sugars. This sugar is absorbed into the bloodstream and causes a spike in the levels of glucose. The body starts producing insulin to counteract the rise in glucose levels.

Insulin is a fat storing hormone and is secreted by the pancreas. When insulin is produced in large amounts, it stops the body from burning fat and all the fat is stored in the body cells. After a while, the body assumes that there is a shortage of essential nutrients and it causes hunger pangs and cravings for all sorts of carb and sugar-rich foods. This means that you will want to eat again, and this vicious cycle keeps going on and on. So, when you restrict your carb consumption, your blood sugar levels will stabilize and this reduces the need for insulin. Instead, it leads to the burning of fats for providing energy and leads to fat loss.

Glucose is favored by the body over fats and it is stored in the liver. However, only a finite amount of glucose can be stored there. The rest is stored in the form of fat, and the storage space for fats isn't restricted. This just leads to the accumulation of fatty cells. When you restrict your carb consumption, the production of glucose reduces as well, and the body will automatically shift to the next available source of energy- fat! Low carb and high-fat diets like the keto diet make it easy for the body to reach into its fat reserves for providing energy. Since these fat reserves aren't blocked by excess insulin, you will start feeling fuller as well. Even when you eat to your heart's content on a keto diet, your calorie intake is bound to reduce. So, you don't have to worry about calorie counting!

Remember that on a keto diet, carbs are limited. So, instead of trying to watch the fats you consume, be mindful of the carbs you eat. Bread, pasta, rice, potatoes, and all other starchy foods should be avoided to achieve ketosis.

The keto diet is a high-fat and a low-carb diet. Since the Mediterranean diet also encourages the consumption of healthy fats and controls carb intake, combining these diets is quite easy. The principle of the keto diet is rather simple. You merely need to eat fats to burn all the stored fats in your body. The keto diet often leads to an imbalance in the level of fats you consume. In fact, you end up concentrating so much on the macros you consume that you can easily forget about the micros you consume while on the keto diet. Ideally, while following the keto diet, you must ensure that about 65-70% of your total calorie intake is in the form of dietary fats, while about 25% comes from proteins and the rest from carbs. On a keto diet, your body shifts its primary source of fuel from burning glucose to burning fats to store energy. This shift is known as ketosis - hence the name of this diet. To achieve ketosis, you will need to restrict your carb intake or even eliminate carbs from your meals.

The combination of the keto diet with the Mediterranean diet is quite brilliant. To combine these two diets, you merely need to eliminate all carbs while drastically reducing your intake of sugars. Apart from this, you can follow all the protocols of the Mediterranean diet.

Intermittent Fasting

Intermittent fasting, as mentioned earlier, alternates

between periods of eating and then fasting. This diet doesn't have any dietary restrictions. Instead, it focuses on the time frame within which you are allowed to eat. There are several methods of intermittent fasting. You might have never consciously thought about it. However, all of us end up fasting daily. Think about it - when you are sleeping, you are fasting. Think of intermittent fasting as a mere extension of this fasting period. You can skip having your breakfast and instead have your first meal at noon and the last one at 8 P.M. This would imply that you will be fasting for about 16 hours daily and the eating window is restricted to a period of 8 hours. This is the most popular method of intermittent fasting and is referred to as the 16/8 method.

Despite what people usually think, this is a very easy schedule to follow. Hunger isn't difficult to manage and tackle. It might be a little difficult initially, however with time it does get easier. You aren't allowed to eat anything during the fasting period. A few beverages like tea and coffee are certainly allowed, but in moderation. There are a couple of different forms of intermittent fasting that allow you to eat low-cal foods in small amounts during the fasting period, as well. Supplements that won't add any additional calories are also allowed.

The concept of fasting isn't a new one, and human beings have been doing this for a long time. It could have been done out of necessity or due to the lack of food. There are religious reasons for fasting, too. Various religions like Islam, Hinduism, Buddhism, and Christianity talk about fasting. Animals and human beings alike tend to fast when they fall sick. There isn't anything that is unnatural or unusual about fasting, and our bodies have been designed in such a way that they can go for long periods of time without any food. Different processes in our bodies also change when we start fasting. The level of blood sugar, as well as insulin, tends to drop down while fasting, and there is an increase in the production of the growth hormone in the body. People follow intermittent fasting since it allows them to shed weight, and it is quite an easy way to achieve that goal. Others follow this diet for the metabolic benefits that it has to offer. There is some research that suggests that this diet can help in providing some protection against diseases that affect the heart and the brain. Intermittent fasting seems like a handy tip that will make your life much simpler, and improve your health simultaneously. The fewer meals you have to plan, the easier your life will be.

Intermittent fasting might mean different things for different people. The most common form of this diet is the 5:2 model. In this, the individual will have to fast for two nonconsecutive days in the week. The rest of the days, there is no restriction on the number of calories that you can consume. There are others who might fast daily and have a fasting window that fits in their schedule. In the 16/8 method, you must fast for about 16 hours in a day and restrict the eating window to about 8 hours. If you want to follow the 24-hour fasting model, you must ensure that you fast for 24 hours at a stretch once a week and eat like you normally do on the other days of the week.

Fasting has many benefits to offer that go well beyond weight loss. Fasting can help in improving your overall health and increase the longevity of your life as well. Some studies examining the link between cell metabolism and fasting found that fasting periodically can help in decreasing the risk of heart diseases, diabetes, aging, and so on. Fasting is effective because, during this period, a lot of cells that are present in the body die and the stem cells start working. This starts the regeneration process and produces new cells. Other studies also show that it helps in reducing the amount of bad cholesterol, or LDL, present in the blood.

If you want to combine the Mediterranean diet with intermittent fasting, then you merely need to select a time window and ensure that the food that you eat during the eating window belongs to the list of items prescribed by the Mediterranean diet. As long as you do this, you will be able to attain the benefits of both of these diets. For instance, if you decide to opt for the 16:8 method, then you must ensure that you are fasting for 16 hours a day. So, if you start fasting at 8 P.M., your fast will go on until noon on the following day. You can break your fast with the first meal at noon. So, this meal that you consume must be something that you will eat while following the protocols of the Mediterranean diet. Yes, it is as simple as that!

Chapter Four: Benefits of the Mediterranean Diet

With dozens of studies supporting the same conclusion, there is no doubt that the Mediterranean diet is one of the world's healthiest eating habits. Of course this did not happen by a stroke of luck.

Researchers have identified four factors that determine a healthy lifestyle namely, a low-fat diet, moderate to no drinking at all, increased physical activity and non-smoking.

In terms of diet, traditional Mediterranean diet definitely has it all. Research has proven that the kinds of foods in this diet have a lot of benefits for your health.

People under this diet have less chances of contracting metabolic illnesses.

The same people also have less chances of getting inflamed cells which reduces the chance of getting disease as well.

Apart from less chances of coronary heart disease and other similar diseases, the Mediterranean diet also lowers the chances of getting other diseases. People in this diet can rest easy knowing that they have a smaller risk of getting cancer. The same thing can be said about Parkinson's and Alzheimer's disease. Equally important is that people in this diet to live longer as well.

Mediterranean Diet and Bone Health

Healthy bones are essential to your long term health and wellness. Bones give your body structure, protect your organs, allow you movement and stability and anchor your muscles and tendons. Most research has shown that a diet strong in calcium, phosphorus and vitamin K before the age of 20 will help to lay down healthy bone. However, there are also other things you can do in mid-life to protect the health of your bones. Eating a Mediterranean style diet is one of those things.

When you don't eat correctly or get enough exercise your bones can weaken and break. These broken bones are painful and may require surgery to correct. Sometimes these weakened and broken bones can cause permanent damage to your ability to be independent for the remainder of your life.

Research published as far back as 2004 shows that there is an association between eating a Mediterranean style diet and an improvement in bone quality. In a study published by the Department of Clinical Epidemiology from the University of Porto Medical school, researchers found that those individuals who followed a Mediterranean diet low in dairy products experienced better bone health than those who ate diets higher in dairy products but not high in fruits, vegetables and monounsaturated fats.

However, when you begin eating a diet rich in vegetables, fruits and monounsaturated fats is important. In Osteoporosis International researchers found that elderly people who started this nutritional plan after the age of 67 didn't experience a decreased risk of fractures. The results of another study found that the elderly experience an increase in serum osteocalcin concentrations after eating a Mediterranean diet, which suggested there were some protective effects on the bone.

Protection against bone loss and breakage during your old age can increase the likelihood that you'll stay home and not be confined to a wheelchair and nursing home. Unfortunately, hip fractures in the elderly can lead to a complete loss of independence without the ability to return to a previous level of activity. Osteoporosis can also result in breaks of the wrist or spine.

Small changes in your dietary habits can improve your bone health and reduce your weight. Foods that are high in monounsaturated fats - like avocados, olive oil, walnuts and seeds - are tasty, increase your feeling of fullness and reduce your overall appetite. These foods are also high in vitamins and essential nutrients for your body.

The standard Western diet is high in refined carbohydrates and white flour, neither of which help to protect the health of your bones or your overall health. The Mediterranean diet is rich in vegetables, fruits, nuts, seeds and plant based oils - a completely different nutritional base than the Western diet. These higher fat foods will stabilize your blood sugar, reduce your risk of diabetes and improve your overall health.

Mediterranean Diet and Cognitive Impairment

Loss of cognition, or the process of acquiring new knowledge and understanding your environment through thought, experience and your senses, can be an extraordinary blow to family members. Cognitive process are both conscious and nonconscious.

The definition of cognitive processes includes the ability to reason, learn, perceive, intelligence and several other capabilities expected of the human mind.

Unfortunately, as people age we expect their cognitive functioning to decline. In fact, up until a couple of decades ago, Alzheimer type symptoms of dementia were almost expected in elderly people. It was expected that people lost their ability to reason, learn and interact appropriately with their environment. But in the past several decades science has learned that the decline of mental abilities is not something that should be expected. Rather, it more likely a function of changing dietary habits from an increase in processed foods, and an increase in the toxic load on our bodies from an increasing number of insecticides and pesticides in our foods.

However, there is hope. Multiple research studies have shown that eating a Mediterranean diet will contribute to the prevention of a series of different brain diseases, associated with a slower cognitive decline and lower risk of Alzheimer's disease and appear to protect against cognitive decline with age.

Another study compared the high healthy fat

Mediterranean diet against the popular low fat diet common in standard Western medicine. Researchers assessed over 500 participants and adjusted for age, education, sex, smoking, physical activity, BMI, hypertension, diabetes, hypertension and a number of other variables. They found that using a diet high in extra virgin olive oil or nuts will would help to improve cognitive function as compared to the use of a low fat diet.

As part of the Nurses Health Study, researchers evaluated the health and dietary habits of over 10,000 women in their late 50s and early 60s and then 15 years later.

They found that those who had better dietary habits in mid-life, eating a Mediterranean type diet, had more healthy aging. They defined health aging as having achieved the age of 70 with no major chronic disease and no major impairment in cognition, mental health or physical function.

Maintaining your cognitive function can increase the potential that you'll remain at home during your retirement years, that you'll find enjoyment in your life and that you'll be able to appreciate and enjoy your friends and family.

Mediterranean Diet and Diabetes

Diabetes is a metabolic disorder in which the body no longer utilizes insulin correctly. There are two different types. One of which the body doesn't make enough insulin or stops altogether, often related to a viral infection or other attack on the pancreas. The second is called type-2 diabetes in which the body makes enough insulin but the cells have developed a resistance to the hormone.

Insulin is responsible for moving glucose or sugar from the bloodstream into the cells to be used for energy. However, the body burns fats for fuel more efficiently, which also reduces the problems with insulin resistance. The standard Western diet is high in carbohydrates and simple sugars, which spike blood sugar and trigger a large release of insulin from the pancreas.

The release of insulin will drop the blood sugar rather quickly, under normal circumstances, which leaves the person feeling a bit shaky and hungry. They often feel cravings for more carbohydrates, which sets up the whole vicious cycle all over again. The release of insulin in large amounts on a daily basis will increase the resistance to the hormone at the cellular level. This is one way that diabetes is triggered.

The Mediterranean diet is often low in carbohydrates, high in vegetables, nuts, seeds and oils. These higher fat foods will keep you feeling full longer, reduce the amount of insulin secreted in the body and level your blood sugar numbers if you already suffer from diabetes.

Your diet and nutrition are crucial tools in the management of the disease. Weight loss can also help to reduce insulin resistance in the body because belly fat or visceral fat found in the abdominal cavity will increase resistance to insulin. When you lose the weight you'll reduce resistance and therefore have better control over your blood sugar levels.

One study published in Diabetes Care from the American Diabetes Association, found that the Mediterranean diet was effective in the prevention of diabetes in people who were already at high risk for cardiovascular disease. Interestingly, these results occured in the absence of any real changes in body weight or increase in physical activity.

In another study published in the same journal 3 years later, researchers found that patients who were newly diagnosed with type 2 diabetes had better reduction in their hemoglobin A1C measurements and had a higher rate of reducing or eliminating their need for insulin when they ate a Mediterranean diet.

A prospective research study published in the British medical Journal found that people who adhered to a Mediterranean diet would reduce their risk of developing diabetes. The researchers followed over 13,000 university graduates without diabetes from Spain for over 4 years.

In a follow-up of a subgroup of this study, researchers found that there was long-term evidence that eating a Mediterranean diet rich in extra virgin olive oil had substantial reduction in the risk of developing diabetes.

Restricted Amounts of Processed Foods and Sugar

As I have already mentioned, the Mediterranean diet is a predominantly plant-based diet and consists of unprocessed foods. This diet is all about the locally available produce as well as organic animal products. The average diet of an American is full of preservatives, sugars, and carb-laden treats as well as different flavor enhancers. The Mediterranean diet is quite different from the diet of an average individual that's filled with convenience foods. A Mediterranean diet is typically low in sugar and barely consists of any artificial ingredients. In fact, this diet encourages its followers to consume small portions of fruits for dessert instead of binging on calorie-rich treats like ice creams, chocolates, or sodas.

Apart from all the plant-based foods, this diet also encourages the consumption of locally caught fish. It also encourages the consumption of goat, sheep, or cow cheeses in small quantities as well as other foods rich in natural fats. Since this diet places emphasis on produce that is locally produced and prohibits the consumption of processed foods, this diet is naturally quite healthy. In fact, reducing the consumption of processed foods and replacing them with healthy and whole foods will make it easier for you to attain your health, weight loss, and fitness goals quite easily.

Lose Weight

Do you want a diet that will help you lose weight while allowing you to eat to your heart's content? Do you want a diet that not only helps with weight loss but also allows you to maintain the weight loss? If yes, then the Mediterranean diet is the best fit. This diet is not only easy to follow, but it is sustainable in the long-run as well. This diet encourages the consumption of foods that are nutrient-dense. Eating this way helps in weight loss as well as the maintenance of the weight loss.

The Mediterranean diet is quite lenient and it does allow some scope for interpretation. Regardless of whether you are interested in following a low-carb, high-protein, or any other form of diet, this diet is a great fit for everyone. It encourages the consumption of foods that are full of naturally healthy fats and reduces the intake of carbs while increasing the intake of proteins. Naturally fatty and healthy oils that consist of Omega-3 along with fibrous foods will leave you feeling fuller for longer. If you're full, then the likelihood of hunger pangs leading to unhealthy snacking is reduced. Not just this, it also helps with portion control without needing any conscious effort.

Take a moment and think about it. If you were to choose between a bowl of salad with a portion of protein and a bar of chocolate, which one do you think will fill you up? Even if the number of calories present in both of these foods is the same, it is obvious that the bowl of salad will fill you up. If you end up eating a bar of chocolate, it is quite likely that you will end up feeling hungry within no time. Not only is your body not getting any nutrition from it, but it also increases your calorie intake unnecessarily.

Plant-based foods are high in fiber, and food that's high in fiber will leave you feeling fuller for longer. This, in turn, helps regulate the portion size of your food without having to pay any conscious thought to it. When you add all this up, it directly leads to a reduction in the number of calories you consume. If you want to lose weight, then you must maintain a calorie deficit. Only when your body burns all the glucose present within will it reach into its internal reserves of fat. To enable your body to do this, you must reduce your calorie intake. So, with the help of the Mediterranean diet, you will be able to reduce your calorie intake without having to worry about hunger pangs or starvation. Not just that, your body will also get all the nutrition that it needs to function optimally. So, it is a win-win through and through.

Lowering Heart Disease

The Mediterranean diet is one of the best alimentary diet for taking the correct intake of omega 3.
The fish oils are rich in Omega -3 fatty acids like EPA and DHA and are found to reduce the level of triglycerides in our body. Having elevated triglyceride levels is a reason for heart diseases. Consuming fatty fish regularly, at least thrice a week will help in getting two important forms of omega 3 fatty acids, called eicosapentaenoic acid (EPA) and docosahexaenoic acid (DHA).
These fatty acids will help in reducing the inflammation and thereby prevent heart disease. People who are suffering from coronary heart disease are advised to take more quantities of fatty fish to prevent artery blockage and blood clotting.
You should be going for a diet that is low in saturated fat and rich in monounsaturated and polyunsaturated fats to

prevent heart diseases. Fish oil has been shown to reduce the problems of irregular heartbeats or arrhythmias. It is very effective in reducing the risk of stroke and also helps in effectively treating the narrowing and hardening of the arteries.

If you take fish oil supplements regularly after you have had a first heart attack, then the risk of getting another heart attack is greatly reduced. It will also help in reducing total mortality and sudden death in patients who have a history of heart diseases.

It will also help in preventing atrial fibrillation in men and women who have undergone coronary artery bypass surgery. DHA rich omega 3 fatty acids will help in reducing the risk of peripheral arterial disease that is associated with chainsmokers.

Taking foods that are rich in higher concentrations of EPA and DHA reduces the risk of nonfatal myocardial infarction in women. Consumption of fatty fish will help in reducing the chances of stroke in elderly people.

Fish oil improves endothelial function in peripheral arterial diseases and also has an amazing effect on blood viscosity for the people who suffering from peripheral vascular disease. The Omega-3 fatty acid that is rich in docosapentaenoic acid (DPA) will help in reducing the risk involved in peripheral arterial disease seen in smokers.

Good, Better, Best

When it comes to fats, people tend to think that these are all bad but this idea could not get any worse. Saturated fats come from animal products while polyunsaturated fats are produced from plants, seeds and vegetable oil among others.

Monounsaturated fats are considered the healthiest and ideally should be included in your diet in place of other kinds of fat.

The good news is that the Mediterranean diet revolves around this line of thinking. Of course it is by no coincidence that this is the reason for the health benefits you get from it. All this is thanks to the kind of staple foods included in all of Mediterranean cuisine.

Foods for Vitality

Mediterranean cuisine takes root from several countries each with its own distinct flavor. At the heart of these dishes though are certain foods that have been proven by research to be important for good health. These foods for vitality are responsible for all the benefits of the Mediterranean diet and making you feel better at the same time.

The following foods are more or less a staple in any Mediterranean dish. You will find them in most recipes no matter what country from the region they come from.

Vegetables

No healthy diet is complete without a serving of vegetables. The truth is that you never have too much vegetable in your diet. For better results, you want to make them part of your lunch and snacks as well. Apart from side dishes on your dinner plate, adding vegetables to your sandwiches can be very tasty as well. Essential vitamins and minerals can be found in vegetables which are important for good health.

Legumes

Legumes are pulses are an important part of any healthy diet. In botanical terms, legumes refer to a certain species of plant. However, it is also used to describe fruits that develop seeds in a pod. These are great sources of fiber and protein.

Fruits and Nuts

Instead of munching on sugary sweets and other junk foods, a much healthier alternative would be to include fruits in your snacks.

Fresh fruits and vegetables contain a variety of minerals, nutrients and vitamins that can help the body function in its maximum potential. Furthermore, the vitamins and nutrients aid in initiating weight loss.

Fruits and vegetables contain antioxidant properties which combat the free radicals. If you adopt the Mediterranean weight loss diet, put more emphasis on the dark leafy green vegetables and include then in virtually every meal.

As such, it is important to stock up on apples, pears and oranges to always have something healthy to eat. Drinking fresh juice is alright but eating an actual piece is a whole lot better.

Nuts on the other hand have calories and contain good monounsaturated fats at the same time. Still, these are better taken in moderation.

Cereals and Grains

Whole grains are good for the health but making the transition from white and processed starches may be difficult for some. For better results, start with whole wheat breads from the lighter variety.

Work your way up to whole grain breads once you get the hang of it. Using this kind of bread for your sandwiches paves the way for a healthy and delicious snack.

Other healthier alternatives include whole wheat pasta which goes with just about any kind of sauce you can think of. It is the same story with brown rice as well. This increases your fiber intake easily. Consider replacing potatoes with sweet potatoes or yams as well.

Cereals which are less processed should be your top choice with oatmeal as the best example. Less sugar and more fiber is the way to go here.

Fish

The Mediterranean diet calls for less servings of red meat and more fish in its place. With fish, you get a good source of protein without having to worry about getting bad fat like in beef and pork. In fact, you get the good kind of fat from fish with Omega-3 fats being the most important among them.

Studies have proven that Omega-3 fats help reduce the risk of heart disease. The progression of such a condition may also be prevented by eating fish or shellfish. Another thing is that fish is relatively more affordable and obviously a healthier source of protein than red meat.

Dairy

Traditional Mediterranean diet does not put a lot of emphasis on dairy products. In fact, people on this diet tend to reduce their consumption of dairy products. Even then, small servings usually of yoghurt and cheese are made occasionally.

Meats

Like dairy, a Mediterranean diet calls for less meats. It is recommended to eat red meat just once a week with the average consumption of only four ounces per day. When choosing meats look for cuts that are leaner since these will have lesser amounts of saturated fats.

Red Wine

People who live in the Mediterranean region love taking wine, in fact, they incorporate wine in their meals especially dinner. Therefore, you should take a moderate amount of wine, especially red wine. Moreover, red wine contains antioxidant properties and can reduce blood clotting thus elevating the risk of strokes. Experts are of the opinion that drinking red wine can reduce the risk of cardiovascular diseases.

Alongside the aforementioned foods to eat in a Mediterranean diet, make sure that you spice up your food with natural and beneficial herbs such as turmeric. Such spices make the food tasty and contain properties and nutrients that can promote your health. Knowing what foods to eat in the Mediterranean diet will definitely help you to make healthy food choices.

Oil in Mediterranean Diet

Olive oil is a type of fat extracted from the olive tree which is a traditional tree from the Mediterranean basin. It is produced by crushing whole olive fruits before the oil is extracted by either chemical or mechanical procedures. Olive oil is used in the cosmetics industry, pharmaceuticals and even in the making of soaps besides cooking.

Olive oil exists in a variety of grades depending on processing. For instance, extra virgin olive oil is considered the premium type. It is produced from the first crushing of olive fruits and is extracted through cold- pressing whereby no chemicals are added. Virgin oil is the second variety, obtained from the second pressing of the fruits and is considered the second-best type. Refined olive oil is obtained from refined virgin olive and it has an acidity level of over 3.3%.

The health benefits of olive oil are wide, a reason why it has been named the Mediterranean miracle. One of its main benefits is that it protects the body against skin, colon and breast cancer. The oil contains phenolic antioxidants, terpenoid and squalene which are all anti- cancer compounds. The oil also has oleic acid which prevents chronic inflammation besides reducing the damage that free radicals cause to body cells.

Olive oil also reduces incidences of type 2 diabetes. This is because the oil has monounsaturated fats like those found in seeds and nuts. These fats are essential in reducing risks of chronic diseases such as diabetes and cancer. A Spanish study that was published in scientific journal diabetes care indicated that any Mediterranean diet which has olive oil is capable of reducing type II diabetes by over 50%.

The oil may be used to significantly reduce osteoporosis. This is a type of infection
which causes reduction in the mass of bones, putting people at a risk of fractures. A test carried out on rats indicated that olive oil increases amounts of phosphorous, calcium and nitrates in the blood, which results in improved thickness of bones to reduce occurrence of the disease.

Blood pressure can significantly be balanced through intake of sufficient amounts of olive oil. Research indicates that it is essential in reducing both diastolic and systolic blood pressures. It is helpful to people taking a diet rich in high amounts fat, whereby three ounces of the fluid each day significantly lower the blood pressure.

The amount of good and bad cholesterol in the body can be controlled by olive oil. The cholesterol considered as bad to the body is LDL, which can be controlled by olive oil because it contains the monounsaturated fats. The oil will also increase the amounts of HDL cholesterol, which is considered the best type of cholesterol in the body.

Olive oil has also been said to control depression. A Spanish study revealed that people who take hydrogenated fats that are mainly found in processed food substances had a 48% risk of suffering depression. In the study, olive oil controlled the risk of cardiovascular attacks, which share a common cause with depression, related to dietary plans hence inclusion of olive oil in the diet can greatly control the two.

So in essence this is an essential type of oil which is recommended for use instead of animal fats such as butter, where possible.

The Bottom Line

The health benefits from the Mediterranean diet all boils down to one thing. All the foods mentioned earlier are rich in essential vitamins and minerals that the body needs for vitality. Consuming these foods can more or less guarantee that you are getting enough of these nutrients. Some of these are the following:

Antioxidants – These help fight off free radicals which are chemical substances that roam around the body and cause damage to the cells.

Carotenoids – This substance is found in red, orange and yellow plants, fruits and flowers. They help protect the body from damage caused by light and oxygen.

Monounsaturated Fats – Also known as the good fat, this can help delay or reduce the risk of heart attack. Studies have also shown that cancer development is lowered as well.

Phytochemicals – These substances can be found mostly in plants and are used for protection against bacteria, viruses and fungi.

Apart from reducing the risk of a wide range of chronic diseases, these are proven to promote longer and healthy living as well.

Chapter Five: The Mediterranean Way of Life

Apart from the food you eat, the Mediterranean diet calls for certain changes in your lifestyle. All this is to live a healthier and longer life. Compared to the American way of life, the Mediterranean one seems harsh and very stressful with little to none of the conveniences you are used to.

In a twist of fate, the Mediterranean way of life is much healthier then the American one. The modern life it seems is responsible for much of the health problems of today.

Of course it is very much possible to live a healthier lifestyle. All it takes is a little planning and adjustments where needed.

Move More, Live More

Physical activity has always been part of the Mediterranean way of life. People have to exert a lot of effort just to grow, harvest and prepare food. This more than fulfills the exercise requirement for a healthier lifestyle.

 It is not even seen as a requirement, just something that has to be done. This is in stark contrast to the American way of life and how exercise is seen as something expendable from the list of daily activities.

Numerous studies have shown that even the simplest forms of exercise can improve your overall health. In an issue of the New England Journal of Medicine published in 1999, it was revealed that women who got regular exercise reduced their risk of a heart attack by as much as 40 percent. Walking for at least five hours a week cuts this risk in half as well. Even exercises lasting only ten minutes of three times a day can have a significant impact.

Exercise has other benefits as well. Old people who undergo an aerobic exercise program will have better mental fitness than those who do not. Studies have proven that old people who exercised reacted 25 percent faster than people who do stretching and toning exercises.

The benefits of exercise to the body are no coincidence. Science has proven that inactivity can result in more risk to chronic diseases including heart disease, cancer diabetes and osteoporosis. The risk for obesity is reduced as well. Getting regular exercise also means better sleep, a more positive outlook and better overall health.

Moving more means preventing high blood pressure and even lowers already high levels of it. It strengthens the heart making it work more efficiently.

At the same time, exercise prevents the spread of chemicals that promote atherosclerosis. With exercise, the body is better able to metabolize carbohydrates and increases sensitivity to insulin. This in turn lowers the incidence of diabetes.

With all these benefits, it comes as no surprise that exercise promotes a longer life. Studies have proven that even the smallest amount of exercise drops mortality rate significantly. This is why an increasing number of physicians prescribe exercise for avoiding chronic diseases.

A Herculean Effort

With the rigorous activity demanded by farming, most Mediterranean folk get their weight training exercise from this. It may not be the same as the weights at the gym but it does have the same effect of strengthening your body.

This includes lifting, hauling, pulling, pushing, loading, chopping and digging among others. Evidently, strength training can become part of daily life without having to go to the gym.

Strength training is somewhat different from other forms of exercises. For one thing, it needs less endurance and more short-term effort of increasing intensity. This builds both muscle and bone structures within the body.

Strong muscles do not just look better, they work better as well. Of course this does not mean huge and hulking muscles. It means muscles that are fit, well-nourished and active.

Bigger muscles are better at processing oxygen which takes some load of the heart. Strong muscles around the joints also help relieve pressure around them. This added strength can certainly make a difference in daily life.

No Time for the Gym?

"No time for the gym" is an excuse you will often hear from people with busy lives. But is this really the case? With so much benefit from exercise, why not spare a few minutes of your time to get up and get going? Even the smallest of things can have a significant impact on your health. Here are a few tips on fitting exercise into your busy schedule:

Shorter but more frequent exercise sessions can be as effective as one entire session. The important thing here is to keep track of the total time and amount of effort exerted.

Skip the elevator and climb up or down the stairs as often as possible. This is a great and simple way to get your heart pumping.

To walk more, park your car as far as possible from your destination. This saves a lot of time and gas circling the parking lot for a convenient space.

Do as much walking as possible. Surely going to the neighbor's house or the grocery does not need a car. When commuting, get off at least two stops earlier and continue the rest of the way on foot.

In the office, get off your chair every fifteen minutes and stretch your muscles. A better idea would be to walk around the office for three minutes.

If you keep missing exercising in the morning, try it in the afternoon instead. Some people are more energetic at that time of the day.

Take your children or your dog to the park to play. How about a quick game of Frisbee while you are at it? This is definitely one of the simplest ways to exercise while having fun with your loved ones.

In the same manner, try to convince a friend to exercise with you. This creates a support system prominently featured in the Mediterranean lifestyle.

Instead of hiring someone else, consider doing your own household chores. Apart from getting exercise, you save money at the same time.

Planning Your Exercises

The American College of Sports Medicine recommended exercise of at least thirty minutes a day most days of the week. This applies for everyone regardless of age and fitness level. For losing weight, aerobic activity of up to sixty minutes a day and strength training are needed.

It may sound too much but it is possible to fulfill this requirement with an exercise plan in place. This plan is quite simple and does not require any special skills, bulky gym equipment or special instruction.

Keep in mind that this is just a guide. The plan calls for exercise for three times a day but you can perform a version for everyday use. You have a free hand at adjusting the intensity level according to what suits you best. In terms of intensity though, be sure that you are working a sweat but not so hard to avoid straining your muscles.

Day One

Perform gentle stretching of up to five minutes. To start your day, perform fifty jumping jacks or start with five first and work your way up to fifty.

Get some fresh air and take a brisk walk for ten minutes during your coffee break.

At lunch, take a brisk walk again for fifteen minutes.

Climb up or down a flight of stairs before dinner.

End the day with as many sit-ups and push-ups as you can add a few repetitions weekly. Finish off with some gentle stretching.

Day Two

This time, walk in place briskly for five minutes but not before some gentle stretching.
Commute to work but get off one stop earlier and walk the rest of the way. This should give you at least ten minutes.
Walk around for fifteen minutes and eat a light lunch.
For your coffee break, stair climbing would be nice.
Finally, ride your bike around before dinner or do something else with equal intensity.

Day Three

Start the day with gentle stretching and continue with five minutes of dancing.
Take a brisk walk for twenty minutes with a few coworkers if possible.
Instead of taking coffee, take two minutes to jog in place then perform ten jumping jacks and twenty wall push-ups. After this regimen, you will not need coffee anymore.
More brisk walking for fifteen minutes wait once you get home after a light dinner. Why not take the whole family with you?
If you have dumbbells or heavy cans of food, use this as weights against your chest while doing some sit-ups.

Portion control

If you want to lose weight, then you must ensure that you are not only following the diet but are also exercising some portion control. Here are a couple of essential portion control guidelines that will come in handy while preparing your meals.

One portion of cooked whole-grain pasta (one serving) is about half a cup - it is almost as big as a hockey puck. One serving contains about 70 calories. One serving of dairy or protein contains about 110 calories. So, about 2/3rd cup of cottage cheese is equivalent to the size of four playing dice. One and a half tablespoons of peanut butter has about 90 calories. There are over 40 calories in 7 almonds. The serving size of protein is about 110 calories, and this is equivalent to two ounces of cooked beef, three ounces of fish or two and a half ounces of skinless chicken. The portion size will resemble a small deck of playing cards- it must essentially be the size of your palm. Two cups of raw spinach count as one serving of vegetables. So, keep these simple things in mind if you want to lose weight and maintain weight loss. For weight loss, it is essential that your body stays in a calorie deficit. It essentially means that your calorie expenditure must be more than what you consume. When this happens, your body will start utilizing its internal reserves of fat to generate energy. This, in turn, will help in burning fat and leads to weight loss.

You and Stress

Modern living has a unique set of demands that can put a

lot of stress in one person. Difficulties with finances, social relationships, careers and parenting are among the most common culprits. Over time, these demands develop into chronic stress and fatigue which is bad for the health.

Stress is a natural reaction of the body which is sometimes called the fight or flight response. It is actually a survival mechanism that has helped ancient peoples. It prepares the body to react quickly and get out of harm's way. Instead of dodging saber-toothed tigers though, modern man is presented with new challenges and dangers.

The stress hormones adrenaline and one that releases corticotropin do certain changes in the body. Blood clumps together and plugs a potential wound and stop bleeding. The immune system prepares for trauma and muscles get a dose of blood sugar and stand ready. At the same time, heart rate and breathing increase.

Once the coast is clear, the body returns to normal thanks to cortisol. However, modern man faces so much stress that returning to normal is next to impossible. The result is a long-term condition that exposes the body to heart attacks.

Coping with Stress in the Mediterranean Way

In the Mediterranean way of life, people had plenty of ways to cope with stress. For one thing, social relationships with family and friends were kept strong and often prioritized. Even neighbors offered support for each other in times of need. This kind of close support helps people cope with stress better.

Another thing is that these people are closer to nature than most others. They grow and harvest their food off the land. While there is not much conclusive evidence to suggest that nature reduces stress levels, anecdotal evidence suggests otherwise. There is just something in nature that puts the mind at ease.

Living With (Out) Stress

Too much stress is bad for the health and this is unacceptable. The answer could not be more obvious. You will need to make a few changes in your lifestyle stress to weed out stress.

Moving to the sun-drenched lands of the Mediterranean sounds like a good idea but is not really possible for most. You should know that it is possible to live a stress-free life in this fast-paced world.

Consider the following tips as your guide:

Appreciate your friends more. Try to improve your social relationships by keeping in touch more. Make it a point to ask family and friends their opinions and ideas. Joining support groups, organizations and other such groups is also a good idea.

Meditation relieves stress and it is a good idea to try it. The visualization involved can be enough to put your mind at ease and chase your worries away. Spend as much as ten minutes of your day to clearing your mind through meditation. How about imagining a relaxing stay at a traditional café on Southern France? Perhaps a stroll through the Greek coastline would do it? This is sure to recharge your mind and body and help you relax more.

Step outside and enjoy the sun with the protection of sunscreen of course. Feel the breeze as it passes through gently and quietly. If you must, drive out of the city and towards somewhere with fresh air and enjoy your stay there.

Consider things in context. Each stressful event, no matter what it may be, should be put into perspective. They may be inconvenient and irritating at times but your whole world does not need to come crashing down. Keep in mind that there are just some things you cannot change no matter how hard you try.

Chapter Six: Living Well with the Mediterranean Diet

Making the switch from your routine diet to a healthier one is a lot easier than you think. In this chapter, you will learn more about how to plan meals in the Mediterranean diet.

Keep in mind that this is just a framework to work with. It is by no means a strict meal plan. You are better off following a meal plan that suits your needs so be sure to make one for yourself.

It is very much possible to lose weight under the Mediterranean diet. For better results though, you want to consult your dietician for the best meal plan for this purpose. Remember that this diet calls for increased physical activity as well. You will need time to lie down, rest and relax too.

You will notice that beverages such as alcohol or coffee are not included in this meal plan. These exclusions are based on the Mediterranean meal plan and are considered optional at best. What you drink during meals in entirely up to you. Be sure to base this decision on your current overall health though.

As a healthier alternative, consider making Green Tea part of your diet. This drink has plenty of health benefits for you. Caffeine and alcoholic drinks should be taken in moderation. This is especially true if you are trying to lose weight.

Recipes for the dishes included in this meal plan can be found in the next chapter. When making a meal plan, keep these guidelines in mind:

Enjoy your food - Remember that relishing every flavor of your food is part of the Mediterranean way of life. Beyond good nutrition, eating is a feast for the senses you must enjoy. It is not considered an inconvenient chore but an important part of life.

Watch the servings. - In any diet, it is important for your calorie intake and activity level to breakeven. For weight loss, you want to consume fewer calories and move around more. Of course this is easier said than done in today's lifestyle. Again, it is important to ask for advice from a dietician or other nutrition expert. In this meal plan, it is up to you to adjust serving sizes to meet your needs.

Drink plenty of water. – As much as possible, try to drink at least six to eight glasses of water a day.

Exercise, rest and relax – Apart from the diet itself, what you do in between meals is an important part of the Mediterranean diet. You should spend less time sitting down and more time moving and getting around. Go outdoors and find something to do to cover your exercise. Be sure to get enough rest and relaxation as well.

Time to Get Started

Based on the traditional diet of the Mediterranean regions,

this diet concentrates on the consumption of vegetables, olive oil, legumes, whole grains, fruits, along with some portion of dairy products, fish, and red wine (only in moderation). If you are interested in turning your life around with this brilliant diet and want to reap all the benefits that it offers, then it is time that you start following the diet! As with any new change, it is ideal to introduce it gradually. The average diet of a westerner is quite different from the one that's prescribed by the Mediterranean diet. So, it is ideal to pace yourself as this will help your body and mind get used to this new way of eating. In this section, you will learn about the different things that you can do to get started with this wonderful diet.

Increase the intake of vegetables

You must try to double or maybe even triple the number of vegetables you consume daily. Vegetables are the cornerstone of a traditional Mediterranean diet. A diet that's plant-based is good for improving your overall health and it reduces the risk of several serious illnesses. Not just that, all the fiber and nutrients present in it are good for the optimal functioning of the body. So, if you want to turn your life around, then please stop saying no to vegetables. Are you worried about how you can make this change? Here are a couple of ideas that you can use to start incorporating vegetables into your daily diet.

If you love having omelets for breakfast, then you merely need to add vegetables of your choice to that omelet. You can even have a mixed-vegetable burrito if you want. Shredded vegetables like spinach, carrots, peppers, and onions along with some smashed avocado and hummus can make for a hearty filling for a wrap.

Simply chuck all your favorite vegetables along with some beans of your choice into a pot and make a hearty stew. You can also make a layered vegetable casserole. You can start making it a point to have at least one portion of salad with every meal that you consume. Make a simple dressing of olive oil, cracked black pepper, salt and lemon juice for a zingy addition to the salad. Apart from this, you can make different sauces using vegetables, too. There are several ways in which you can easily incorporate vegetables into your daily life. Go through the delicious Mediterranean diet recipes given in this book for more inspiration.

Start loving legumes

The primary sources of protein in this diet are different types of lentils, peas, and beans. Not only are legumes rich in proteins, but they are full of dietary fibers. For instances, one cup of navy beans has considerably more protein than two whole eggs and more fiber than eight slices of whole-wheat bread. Apart from this, legumes are also a rich source of polyphenol antioxidants as well as resistant starch - a type of starch that is indigestible and helps in improving the functioning of the gut bacteria. It also helps in promoting weight loss and protects the gut from different inflammatory disease. So, you must start adding plenty of legumes to your diet. Here are a couple of ideas that you can use to start incorporating legumes into your daily diet.

You can make a zesty dip by pureeing white beans, red peppers, and garlic. You can add kidney beans to any vegetable stew or soup. Beans are quite versatile, and you can add them to salads and even make vegetable burger patties by grinding them with other vegetables.

Fish and seafood

Fish, as well as any other seafood, is a major part of the Mediterranean diet. They are great sources of lean protein and also have other essential nutrients in them like selenium, Vitamin B, and Vitamin D. Fatty fish are also rich in Omega-3 fatty oils. By including about two ounces of fish to your daily diet, you can considerably reduce the risk of different heart diseases and vitamin deficiencies. Fatty fish like salmon, sardines, tuna, herring, mackerel, and sardines are great sources of Omega-3 fatty acids that help in reducing the risk of cholesterol and other heart conditions. Here are a couple of ideas that you can use to start incorporating fish into your daily diet:

You can bake cod or tilapia with different vegetables like leeks, peppers, olives and herbs. Shrimp skewers served with a portion of salad makes for a wonderful meal. Incorporate tuna or salmon into sandwich fillings. Apart from this, seafood pairs wonderfully with different kinds of pasta.

Change the oil

As I have been mentioning, olive oil is the go-to oil for cooking in Mediterranean cuisine. The high levels of monounsaturated fats present in it help in protecting your body against the threat of cardiovascular dysfunction and heart disease. All that you need to do is simply replace your regular cooking oil with olive oil. You can even add it to salad dressings! The nutty flavor of olive oil pairs wonderfully with pretty much anything that you want to cook.

Start eating fruit for dessert

If you have a sweet tooth and like to have some dessert at the end of every meal, then you must think about replacing dessert with fruit. You can have a portion of fresh or frozen fruit for dessert. For instance, you can blend frozen berries with a tablespoon of yogurt and enjoy some fresh fruity yogurt. You can also have a handful of berries with unsweetened whipped cream. Instead of reaching for a bag of cookies or a scoop of ice cream, have a serving of fruit. Also, fruits make for a great snack.

If you find that you are still hungry after a meal, then you can indulge in a cup of tea or coffee while the rest can finish their sweet treats. Good options would be decaf coffee or herbal tea as well. Stay away from sugar-laden desserts, as these are dense in calories and don't have any nutritional value at all. A good replacement option would be berries and some heavy cream, or you can add in some cream to your coffee for satiating your sweet tooth. Look for different low-fat and low-sugar variations of the desserts you like. You could also add some honey to melons to sweeten them up a little.

Dairy as a garnish

Dairy can help in reducing the risk of metabolic syndromes, cardiovascular diseases, as well as the risk of diabetes. When consumed in small quantities, it can even prevent the risk of obesity. I am not talking about stuffing a sandwich with lots of processed cheese or covering pasta with a thick layer of cheese. The traditional Mediterranean diet includes small quantities of cheese and yogurt - usually made from goat's milk. The best way to add dairy to your diet is by using it as garnish. You can add crumbled feta or goat's cheese to a salad or any other main course. You can also use Greek yogurt for making dressings as well as dips.

Seasonings matter

If you are used to adding extra salt to your food, stop doing that starting today. Don't add extra salt to your salad or your fries. Excess sodium increases your blood pressure and puts extra stress on your heart. It can also have an adverse effect on the functioning of your kidneys and strain them unnecessarily. Salt isn't the only flavoring agent that you can use. Make use of different spices to flavor your food. Use sea salt or rock salt, instead of the refined salt you find in the market.

Spices and herbs don't only lend flavor to the food, but they have several health benefits as well. Garlic, as well as herbs, are the go-to seasonings in the typical Mediterranean cuisine. Unlike American cuisine, which relies on salt for seasoning, the Mediterranean cuisine uses a variety of different seasonings. Did you know that garlic has certain compounds present in it that help in reducing cholesterol while strengthening the function of the immune system? Different herbs like parsley, thyme, oregano and such also contain high levels of antioxidants and other phenolic compounds as well as flavonoids that not only have antibacterial properties, but help in improving the brain's health, too. So, don't hesitate to season your food with Mediterranean spices. Adding certain spices can help in improving your overall health. Cinnamon can be used in sweet and savory foods, and it helps in regulating the blood sugar levels in the body.

Cinnamon behaves like natural insulin. Oregano is a flavorful herb, and it tastes great even when dried. Oregano has plenty of antioxidants and it seamlessly is blended with other flavors. Rosemary helps in reducing inflammation. One of the leading causes for several chronic health conditions like arthritis is inflammation. Adding some rosemary to your food regularly can help in reducing this inflammation. Thyme is full of antioxidants, and it improves the respiratory function. Last but not least, dried red peppers like cayenne pepper help with weight loss.

Reduce your intake of meat

The Mediterranean diet is native to all the regions along the coast of the Mediterranean Sea. This means that the inhabitants' usual diet didn't include a lot of meat - at times due to religious reasons, too. The meat that's used is usually organic and pasture-raised. Such meats have a high level of omega-3 fatty acids as well as conjugated linoleic acid or CLA, that helps in burning fats while improving the overall function of the immune system. So, if you do want to include meat to your diet, I suggest that you opt for the grass-fed or the pasture-raised variants instead of the factory farmed meats. Also, it is a good idea to treat meat like a garnish or a condiment instead of the main ingredient. You can add some portion of grilled meats to a salad or something along those lines. The primary focus of the Mediterranean diet is on seafood and not meats. So, it is time that you slowly start cutting down on the meat that you consume, if you are used to eating a lot of meat.

Include some pasta

Pasta made out of durum wheat is full of natural fibers that prevent any fluctuations in the level of blood sugar in the body. Since it is fibrous food, it takes a while for your body to absorb it, and this means that you will be left feeling fuller for longer. So, before you pick pasta the next time you go grocery shopping, carefully go through the ingredients to avoid picking up any that are made from processed wheat. Always opt for the whole-grain variants and even check out the different gluten-free options that are available these days. To go with pasta, instead of calorie-rich fatty sauces, make sauces full of vegetables and seasonings. The only cheese that you add should be in the form of seasoning. You can always sprinkle grated parmesan or crumbled feta on the pasta.

Enjoy the food

It's a good idea to remind yourself, and those around you, that eating isn't a race. Take the time to savor what you eat and enjoy your food. You are likely to realize when you are full when you start chewing your food more, and it also helps aid digestion. Along the way, you will begin to notice the different flavors in the food that you might have never noticed before. Don't switch on the TV while eating, either, and keep your phone on silent mode. You don't need any distractions while eating. Make your dining room an electronics-free zone. You don't realize what you eat and how much you eat when you are watching TV. Instead, spend the mealtime with your loved ones. This is a great way to get involved in each other's lives and is a nice habit to get into to unwind after a tiring day.

Food Shopping List

Let us take a look at the groceries that you can stock up on so that you can cook a meal on short notice. This section will give you a quick list of vegetables, dairy products, meat & poultry, fruits, beans, fish and more to stock up on for a Mediterranean diet. Having these products handy will ensure that you don't deviate from your diet and eat a healthy Mediterranean meal at all times.

Vegetables

Try to include as many seasonal vegetables as you can. Also, I suggest that you opt for produce that is locally grown. Whenever possible, go for the organic variants instead of the commercially farmed ones. Here is a list of vegetables that you can include in your shopping list:

Tomatoes, bell peppers (yellow, green, and red), onions, eggplant, zucchini, green beans, peas, okra, cucumber, cauliflower, broccoli, garlic, cabbage, lettuce (romaine, iceberg, butterhead), celery, carrots, mushrooms, squash, and beets.

You can also add different greens like spinach, amaranth, beet greens, chicory and any other leafy veggies you can think of.

Dairy products

The dairy products that you opt for must be the full-fat variants and not the "low-fat," "non-fat," or "diet" options. The dairy items you can include are Greek yogurt, ricotta, goat's cheese, yogurt made from sheep's milk, feta cheese, parmesan, cottage cheese, graviera and mizithra.

Meat and poultry

Red meat is usually consumed very infrequently in this diet, and I suggest that you limit it to about once or maybe twice per week and not more than that. Chicken (preferably skinless), veal, ground beef, and pork can be included.

Fats and nuts

Extra virgin olive oil, virgin olive oil, or any other olive oil as long as it is of good quality. Tahini, almonds, walnuts, pistachios, cashews, pine nuts and sesame seeds.

Beans

Different types of legumes are a staple source of protein. So, you can include lentils, yellow split peas, chickpeas, and white beans.

Fish and seafood

Anchovies, sardines, salmon, tuna, mackerel and herring along with shrimp, octopus and calamari can be added to your shopping list.

Fruits

Oranges, tangerines, lemons, apricots, figs, apples, pears, cherries, peaches, cantaloupe and watermelon.

Grains and bread

Whole grain bread, barley rusks, whole grain breadsticks, pita bread, phyllo sheets, wholegrain or gluten-free pasta, rice, bulgur and couscous.

Herbs and spices

Oregano, parsley, dill, mint, basil, cumin, allspice, cinnamon, pepper, sea salt and paprika.

Pantry staples

Canned tomatoes, olives, tomato paste, capers, balsamic vinegar, red wine vinegar, olives, sun dried tomatoes, honey and some wine.

Planning Your Meals

This sample meal plan outlines the typical foods you eat under the Mediterranean diet. It covers the three main meals and one snack per day for a whole week. Keep in mind that this is just a rough guide to help you get started. Feel free to add and remove items to fit your individual needs.

Sunday

<u>Breakfast</u>
A serving of Frittata made of 1 egg, 2 egg whites and ½ cup of sliced portabella mushrooms, 1 teaspoon of dill and ¼ cup of skim milk or water then mixed together and cooked with olive oil
1 to 2 slices of whole-grain toast
1 cup of low-fat and calcium-fortified soy milk
<u>Lunch</u>
A serving of Mediterranean Vegetables with Walnuts and Olive Vinaigrette
½ cup of White Beans with Cumin
1 small whole-grain roll
<u>Snacks</u>
A serving of Broiled Tomatoes
<u>Dinner</u>
A serving of Chicken Raisin Stew
A serving of Green Salad and Olive Oil Vinaigrette
½ piece of whole-grain pita pocket and 1 tablespoon of Tapenade

Monday

<u>Breakfast</u>
Eat 1 cup of oatmeal made of whole oats. Try this with fresh blueberry toppings and 1 tablespoon of raw walnuts.
Chow down this meal with 1 cup of low-fat soy milk. Drinking one that is calcium fortified is much better.

Lunch

Eat 1 pita pocket oh whole grain variety and filled with salad greens, 2 to 3 ounces of tuna and some mustard.

1 cup of red grapes

For dessert, try eating 1 cup of nonfat or low-fat yogurt of plain variety. Add 1 teaspoon honey or maple syrup.

Snacks

6 to 12 whole almonds and 1 to 2 whole wheat breadsticks

Dinner

Eat 1 cup of Tuscan Bean Soup with half a cup of brown rice.

2 cups of green salad and tomatoes with 1 tablespoon of Olive Oil Vinaigrette

1 serving of Cinnamon Oranges

Tuesday

Breakfast

2 pieces of small Orange-Banana Muffins

1 ½ cups of low-fat and calcium-fortified soy milk

½ to ¾ cup of berries

Lunch

1 serving of Sweet Corn and Toasted Walnut Risotto

1 serving of Macedonian Salad

Snacks

A serving of baby carrots with 1 to 2 tablespoons of Hummus Tahini

Dinner

A serving of Swordfish Steaks and Tomato-Caper Sauce

A serving of Greek Salad

A serving of Wine-Stewed Figs with Yogurt Cream

Wednesday

<u>Breakfast</u>

1 egg and 2 egg whites scrambled with ¼ cup of skimmed milk, black pepper and fresh herbs

1 slice of whole-grain toast

½ grapefruit

<u>Lunch</u>

A serving of Gazpacho

A serving of Olive Oil Cheese Crisps

1 apple

1 cup of low-fat and calcium-fortified soy milk

<u>Snacks</u>

Caponata served with ¼ whole-grain pita pocket

<u>Dinner</u>

A serving of Ginger Lamb Stew

A serving of steamed broccoli tossed with minced garlic, hot pepper flakes and olive oil

½ cup of nonfat frozen vanilla yogurt with prune puree or berries for toppings

Thursday

<u>Breakfast</u>

1 cup of whole-grain flaxseed cereal

1 cup of low-fat and calcium-fortified soy milk

2 to 4 whole pitted dates or prunes sliced into cereal

<u>Lunch</u>

A serving of Tabbouleh Salad

A serving of Sauteed Shrimp with Chillies

½ cup of pineapple chunks

<u>Snacks</u>

A serving of Broiled Tomatoes

<u>Dinner</u>

A serving of Mediterranean Salad Sandwich with Harissa Stuffed Peaches

Friday

<u>Breakfast</u>

¾ cup of Almond Couscous

½ cup of mandarin oranges

<u>Lunch</u>

A serving of Falafel with Tomato-Cucumber Relish

A serving of Green Salad with shredded carrots and olive oil vinaigrette

1 pear

1 cup of skimmed milk or low-fat and calcium-fortified soy milk

<u>Snacks</u>

A serving of broccoli florets and dipped in 1 teaspoon of olive oil mixed with 1 tablespoon of lemon juice

<u>Dinner</u>

A serving of Mediterranean Citrus Chicken

½ cup of spinach sautéed with 1 teaspoon of olive oil, minced garlic and 1 tablespoon of balsamic vinegar
Slices of apple dipped in 1 tablespoon of almond butter

Saturday

Breakfast
2 flaxseed or whole-grain waffles and sliced banana
1 cup of low-fat and calcium-fortified soy milk
Lunch
A serving of Moroccan-Spiced Cod
A serving of Beet Salad with Walnuts
2 fresh apricots and 1 cup of nonfat plain or sweetened yogurt
Snacks
1 sliced wheat bread with sprouts and 1 teaspoon olive oil
Dinner
A serving of Tuna Steaks with Green Sauce
1 cup of steamed green beans with minced fresh basil and ¼ cup of crumbled feta cheese
1 fresh nectarine

Chapter Seven: Keeping the Weight Off

Losing weight is one thing but keeping the weight off is another. The good news is that you can easily adjust your diet from a weight loss one to a maintenance one. This time, you can eat a wider range of foods. However, it is still best to focus on whole grains, plant foods, whole vegetables and fruits, fresh fish and shellfish, healthy fats and lean proteins.

Keep in mind that the Mediterranean diet is a commitment on your part. Hopefully, your kitchen does not play host to junk foods and other unhealthy snacks anymore. In its place are fresh stocks of food and bottles of olive oil ready to spring into action anytime.

You can always use other similar foods to replace the ones for each item. Feel free to add more fruits, vegetables and whole grains if you still feel hungry. Adjust your portions as necessary. Remember that his is only a guide meant to give you an idea on what to expect. For best results, you want to tailor this meal plan according to your age, weight, height, gender, activity level and overall health.

This makes it very important to seek professional advice from a dietician and other qualified personnel. The goal here is to consume a wide variety of healthy foods as prescribed by the Mediterranean Diet Pyramid. Of course be sure that you enjoy and savor every bite.

The menu listed below is your guide for well-balanced eating. It is meant for neither weight gain nor weight loss. Instead, you will be able to maintain your current weight with this meal plan. This is possible because of the nature of the meal plan in giving you enough energy and making you feel better about yourself.

The serving portions have been intentionally left vague. This is to encourage you to adjust your servings and eating habits according to your own needs. In turn, it is up to you to make sure that you are not eating too much at any time. When this happens though, you can always fall back to the meal plan for weight loss presented earlier.

Sunday

Breakfast
Grapefruit broiled with a sprinkle of brown sugar
1 scrambled egg with 1 ounce cheese topping
2 slices of whole-grain toast
Lunch
A serving of Ratatouille
A serving of white bean tossed in olive oil, fresh or dried basil and fresh lemon juice
Snacks
1 ounce of low-fat cheese and whole-grain crackers
Dinner
A serving of French Cassoulet
A serving of Green salad with Olive Oil Vinaigrette

Homemade custard made using skim milk or low-fat and calcium-fortified soy milk and berries for toppings

Monday

<u>Breakfast</u>
1 to 2 cups of whole-grain cereal with a handful of dried fruit and ½ ounces of dried nuts for toppings
1 cup of low-fat and calcium-fortified soy milk
<u>Lunch</u>
2 slices of whole-grain bread with 3 or more large leaves of Romaine lettuce, 1 ounce part-skim mozzarella cheese, 3 ounces of low-fat turkey breast, a dash of olive oil and a little bit of salt and pepper
1 piece of fresh pear
<u>Snacks</u>
6 to 12 pieces of whole almonds and whole-grain crackers
<u>Dinner</u>
A serving of Moroccan Vegetable Stew
Couscous
A serving of Green Salad and shredded carrots drizzled with Olive Oil Vinaigrette
Fresh berries and ½ cup of soy ice cream in vanilla flavor

Tuesday

<u>Breakfast</u>
Banana bread baked with olive or canola oil and whole-grain flour

½ ounce of nuts or seeds which can be mixed into the bread

1 piece of fresh orange

1 cup of low-fat, calcium-fortified soy milk with vanilla extract and a dash of cinnamon

Lunch

1 cup of pasta mixed with olive oil and topped with ½ ounces of walnut pieces, fresh parsley and 1 tablespoon of grated Parmesan cheese

A serving of Green Salad with Olive Oil Vinaigrette

Stuffed Peaches

Snacks

A serving of baby carrots and Hummus Tahini

Dinner

A serving of Tuscan Bean Soup

A serving of Macedonian Salad

1 to 2 slices of whole-grain bread

½ ounces of low-fat cheese

Wednesday

Breakfast

A serving of oatmeal or other hot cereal mixed with 1 to 2 cups of skim milk to cook and 1 to 2 spoonfuls of pumpkin puree, a tablespoon each of snipped dried apricots, raisins, walnuts and a sprinkling of brown sugar

Lunch

A serving of mashed white beans and whole-wheat pita bread

A serving of Greek Salad

A serving of Citrus Compote

<u>Snacks</u>

1 slice of whole-grain toast and 1 ½ tablespoons of peanut or almond butter

<u>Dinner</u>

A serving of Paella Valencia

A serving of steamed broccoli tossed in olive oil, hot pepper flakes and minced garlic

½ cup of nonfat frozen yogurt with prunes or berries for toppings

Thursday

<u>Breakfast</u>

1 piece of whole-grain bagel and 2 tablespoons of almond or peanut butter

6 pitted dates

1 cup of low-fat and calcium-fortified soy milk

<u>Lunch</u>

A serving of Mediterranean Vegetables and Walnuts and Olive Oil Vinaigrette

½ cup of pineapple slices mixed with ½ cup of plain non-fat yogurt

<u>Snacks</u>

A serving of steamed and chilled green beans dipped in Olive Oil Vinaigrette

<u>Dinner</u>

A serving of vegetable pizza with ½ ounces of part-skim

mozzarella cheese
A serving of Stuffed Artichokes
A serving of Baked Apples and Pears

Friday

<u>Breakfast</u>
1 to 2 cups of whole-grain cereal, ½ ounces of nuts, dried
fruit mixed with 1 cup of plain non-fat yogurt
<u>Lunch</u>
Whole-grain sesame crackers with Tapenade
Green salad with tomatoes, ¼ ounces of sliced almonds and
Olive Oil Vinaigrette
1 tangerine
1 cup of low-fat and calcium-fortified soy milk
<u>Snacks</u>
Broccoli florets with a plain non-fat yogurt blended with
low-fat cottage cheese as dip
<u>Dinner</u>
A serving of Seafood Risotto
½ cup of spinach sautéed in olive oil and mince garlic
A serving of grilled bananas

Saturday

<u>Breakfast</u>

Whole-grain pancakes made with olive oil and non-fat
yogurt with ½ cup of fresh fruit, ¾ cup of nonfat yogurt
and ½ ounces of nuts of your choice as toppings

1 cup of low-fat and calcium-fortified soy milk

Lunch

A serving of Falafel with Tomato-Cucumber Relish

Green salad served with Olive Oil Vinaigrette and fresh plum tomatoes

4 pieces of whole dried apricots

Snacks

1 slice of whole-grain toast with sunflower seeds and peanut butter as toppings

Dinner

Eggplant parmesan

1 cup of Italian green beans and oregano

Fruit salad made with fresh fruits

Healthy snack options

Mediterranean Diet snack options can help you stay healthy and lose weight. Just by making some simple modifications in your regular meal habits, you can have many advantages and the Mediterranean Diet is one of the best solutions to choose.. You can select the following 10 snacks to help you in your nutrition plan:

Dried Apples

According to experts, women who eat dried apples every day can slightly improve their health. The equivalent of 240 calories of dried apples can lower the level of cholesterol 23 percent.

Red Wine

While enjoying your meal, a glass of wine is one of the things that matter, because the drink is full of antioxidants. In order to ensure the drink is beneficial to your body, you should not exceed the recommended amount of one glass per day.

Yogurts

Yogurts are good for the Mediterranean diet, but not all. You must choose only low-fat, or non-fat products. One of the best options to choose is the plain Greek yogurt. In comparison to regular products, Greek yogurts can be tangy, thick & creamy and they contain a lot of proteins.

Pumpkin Seeds

The body makes serotonin from the tryptophan amino acid, which is contained by pumpkin seeds. This substance can help you sleep better and provide a good general mood.

Crackers with Tuna

The type of tuna which should be used is light tuna that is water-packed. Instead of using mayonnaise and other similar dressings, you can use olive oil for flavour, along with spices. You could add some vegetables too and consume the tuna with whole grain crackers.

Fruit Salad

Fruit can be great for dessert with any Mediterranean type of meal. Try to cut different types of fruit and do not forget to add berries, as they have antioxidant properties.

Baked Sweet Potato Fries

Sweet potatoes can be combined with olive oil and they contain carotenoids, which are antioxidant compounds that are known to protect you from cancer, heart diseases and other illnesses. Sweet potatoes can keep your glycemic level low, because of the fibers that they can provide.

Roasted Chickpeas

You could prepare roasted chickpeas with olive oil, paprika and salt. By rinsing, draining and pat drying two cans of chickpeas, you can obtain an awesome snack. The ingredients must be placed on a rimmed baking sheet and they could be drizzled with olive oil. The next step is roasting them into a hot oven for thirty to forty minutes. Salt and paprika must be added in the final roasting minutes.

Pistachios

Also called skinny nuts, pistachios have the lowest number of calories of all nuts. Also, skinny nuts have antioxidants. Overeating is discouraged with these ingredients, because eating them takes longer

Nuts

Nuts are full of nutrients. But, for losing weight, they must be eaten with moderation. Eating not more than ten to twenty nuts at a meal can be the best thing to do. You can find on the market packs of 100 calories and these can be ideal.

Chapter Eight: Common Mistakes to Avoid

To stay on the right track, keep in mind a few mistakes to avoid while following this diet to ensure that it is effective.

The first thing that you must always remember is that weight loss doesn't take place until you maintain a calorie deficit. So, if your calorie intake is too high and there isn't any physical activity, then this diet cannot do you much good. Leading a sedentary lifestyle isn't good if you want to derive the health and physical benefits this diet, or any diet, offers. So, ensure that you exercise at least three times per week. This doesn't necessarily mean you need to do a high-impact workout or spend an hour at the gym. Anything that gets you moving counts.

You must monitor your food intake as well as the portions you consume. As I mentioned, the typical Mediterranean diet doesn't include much meat or cheese since they weren't easily available. Even on the occasions when they were available, they were quite scarce. So, consume these ingredients rarely and in limited quantities. In fact, it is suggested that you limit your consumption of red meats to only once or twice a week.

Always opt for seasonal produce instead of the frozen variants. Try to consume fresh produce. In fact, the ideal modes of cooking are grilling or eating them raw whenever possible instead of frying the ingredients.

Another common mistake that a lot of beginners tend to make is that they load up on bread and pasta. You can certainly include them in your diet, but in limited portions. If you fill yourself up with carbs, it will not do you any good. If you keep providing your body with an endless supply of carbs, whatever leftover glucose produced from them will be stored as fat. So, instead of doing this, it is a good idea to load on up on vegetables and lean animal proteins. Never binge on carb-rich foods.

Olive oil is certainly a major component of the typical Mediterranean diet, but you must consume it in moderation. You can use it for cooking and also in dressings, but ensure that you don't go overboard. Even the healthiest of oils have calories and fat in them. So, while cooking, I suggest that you carefully follow the quantities specified in the recipes given in this book. Do this until you get the hang of how much you must consume.

Also, this diet does allow you to indulge in an occasional glass of wine. Please don't think of this as a license to drink as much as you want. A glass of red wine with your meals is fine if you do it occasionally. Alcohol has plenty of hidden carbs and sugars in it. If you overindulge, you cannot derive the health benefits this diet offers.

The Mediterranean diet is not a low-fat diet. Don't be under any misconception that it is a low-fat diet. In fact, this diet includes plenty of healthy fats, as you are now aware. It is essential that your body gets sufficient healthy fats for it to function optimally. So, don't think that by opting for the low-fat variants, you will be doing your body any good. By eliminating healthy fats, you will prevent this diet from working optimally.

Another common mistake that a lot of people make is that they aren't patient. When you are adopting a new diet, please understand that your body will take some time to get used to it. So, in the meanwhile, you must be patient. It can take over three weeks before you can see a positive change. If you want to see quick results, then you will be disappointed. Give the diet some time to work its magic. In the meanwhile, trust the diet, stick to it, and engage in some physical activity. All of this will lead to a positive change in your overall health.

Chapter Nine: Tips to Stay Motivated

It can be difficult to keep your motivation high when it comes to achieving your weight loss and fitness goals. Why else do you think so many people keep making their New Year's resolution to lose weight but fail to achieve it? Once the novelty of the diet fades away, so does the motivation. Once you lose your motivation, it can become rather difficult to follow any diet. You must learn to be your own cheerleader and think of ways in which you can ensure that your spirits stay high. In this section, you will learn about the different tips that will come in handy to ensure that your motivation doesn't falter while dieting.

Pep Talks Work

Positivity can be contagious. Take a couple of minutes out of your daily schedule and spend this time channeling your inner self. Give yourself a pep talk, tell yourself that you can attain your goals and, essentially, you must allow the positivity to flow. You can even write down some positive affirmations or say them out loud. Use positive affirmations to keep up your spirits.

Set Realistic Goals

If you want to stay motivated when you get started with

your diet, then you must set some realistic goals. You must not only set goals, but you must set goals that are achievable. Before you start dieting, set your goals to define what you wish to achieve by following the diet. Your goals will determine your success in the long-run. If you come up with unattainable or impractical goals, then be prepared to be disappointed. For instance, if your weight loss goal is to shed about 30 pounds in three weeks, you will more than likely end up disappointed. Not only is it impossible to attain, but it is quite unhealthy, too. Did you gain all those extra pounds overnight? I am sure that you didn't, so how can you expect to lose them in no time? So, you must set practical and achievable goals. A reasonable goal is to try and lose one pound per week. This is doable. If you create a sensible pattern of eating and stick to it, you can attain this goal.

Don't Rush

The success of this diet will depend on all the lifestyle changes you are willing to make. This can take some time. If you are interested in losing weight and ensuring that it doesn't come back, then you must pace your weight loss. If you want, you can drastically reduce your food intake and starve yourself to lose weight. However, not only is this manner of weight loss unsustainable, but it is quite harmful to your overall well being. Ensure that your weight loss is gradual and not drastic. The Mediterranean diet is a wonderful option because it allows you to lose weight in a sustainable manner. So please don't be in a rush, and pace yourself instead.

Setbacks are Common

Setbacks are common in all aspects of life. There is no way to predict when some temptation might strike you. At times you will be able to fight it off, and at others you might just give in. This is okay, and it is something that you must accept. The problem only starts when you think of a small setback as a failure. So you gave in and ended up binging on a lot of carbs. If you tell yourself that it is a setback, an isolated incident that you don't plan on repeating, then you will be fine. However, if you start thinking of this as a way to go back to your unhealthy eating habits, then you will find yourself in a world of trouble. Forget about the setback and ensure that you go back to following your diet at the next meal.

Perfectionism is Not Good

The perfectionist attitude of all or nothing will become quite troublesome if you are following a new diet. You don't have to be a perfectionist and, as mentioned setbacks are common. If you don't lose your perfectionist attitude, then you will start thinking of every small obstacle as a failure. All this negativity is bound to take a toll on your mojo sooner or later. So, ensure that you keep a positive attitude while starting a new diet.

Find a Partner

Making a lifestyle change isn't all that easy, and at times it might feel like an uphill battle. Well, you aren't alone in this, and you must know this. You can find people who have similar goals as yours and buddy up with them. Different forums and groups help with dieting. You can join one such group. If you don't want to do so, the next option is to find yourself a dieting partner. You can depend on your dieting partner for some motivation, especially when you feel like giving up. Your dieting partner can be your spouse, a family member, a friend, or even your colleague at work. Your buddy can keep track of your diet and exercise regime with you. When you are accountable to someone else, it improves the chances of your success.

Reward Yourself

Following a new diet is not an easy change to make and it might seem more troublesome than fun at times. So, you must make a reward program for yourself. Whenever you attain a goal, regardless of how small it is, you must treat yourself. Remember that you are your own cheerleader. The rewards you set for yourself must not be related to food. So, if you have attained your weight loss goal for a week, have followed the diet for a week, or maybe exercised three times in a week, feel free to treat yourself. Maybe you can go ahead and buy those shoes you have been eyeing for a while, or how about a spa day? Pamper yourself a little. Also, by creating a reward system, you will be providing yourself with the motivation to keep going.

Maintenance Plan

A lot of people seem to find that it is easier to lose weight than it is to maintain that weight loss. It is quintessential that you realize that your idea of eating healthily isn't just a temporary adjustment and is something that you wish to continue in the long run. It is certainly not a one-time project, and it helps if you keep this in mind. So, create a maintenance plan for the diet if you want to keep the weight off and improve your overall health.

Photograph your Progress

Before you get started, one thing you can do is take a photograph of yourself. This will be the "before" photograph. It will help you in getting started with the diet. If you follow the protocols of this diet, you will find the motivation you need to get through. You can gauge your progress by comparing yourself to that image. This will certainly make you want to keep going. After a while, you will see a positive change in your body. Also keep in mind that it's not about the scale - a healthy body isn't a number, but a feeling.

Eat Healthy Foods First

While eating, start with foods that are rich in nutrients. This is an ideal practice, especially when you are fasting for a longer period. Your body will need nourishment. It isn't the quantity but the quality of food that matters. Nutrition must be your priority. So, have foods that are rich in proteins and natural fats instead of carbs. Not only will this leave you feeling fuller for longer, but it is better for your health as well. Once you fill yourself up with all these foods, you can eat anything else that you want - as long as it is Mediterranean diet-friendly.

Hydrate Yourself

You must ensure that your body is thoroughly hydrated at all times, even when you are following a diet. Water is essential, not just to hydrate your body, but to help flush out any toxins from your system, clear your skin, and keep hunger pangs at a bay. Make it a point to drink at least eight glasses of water daily. Each glass should be 20-ounces. Regardless of what you eat, you must drink water. So, it is a good idea to carry a water bottle with you. To make flavored water, you can add slices of oranges, lime, or sprigs of mint.

Find a Local Farmer

If you cannot find a local farmer, then you can search for a local farmer's market. Instead of buying your meat from a supermarket, opt for these places. The quality is better, and you will be aware of what the animals were fed. Also, the price can sometimes be lower. Buying from a farmer is cheaper than buying from a supermarket, especially if you are buying in bulk. Buying local produce is always healthier, too. Not just that, it is more ethical as well. You can always ask a local farmer to show you around the farm. This will help you in understanding how the food that ends up on your table is being tended to.

Buy Seasonal Produce

If you are purchasing fruits and vegetables from a farmer or a farmer's market, then the produce is bound to be seasonal. If you are picking these up from a supermarket, then you will never learn about seasonal produce. The only indication would be their price. The price of produce at the beginning of their respective season is higher, since not much of it is available. With the advent of globalization, most of the foods we eat can be purchased at any given point in time. Nowadays, the availability of vegetables and fruits isn't restricted to their seasons. You can find tropical fruits and berries throughout the year these days. Not only are out of season fruits and vegetables expensive, but they also lack quality as well. Depending on where you reside, learn a little about the local produce. Make sure that you are buying seasonal produce whenever possible.

Plan your Cooking Well in Advance

Some people are capable of cooking anything with the ingredients available on hand, while others need to make plans to avoid waste. Planning what you will have to cook in advance can be quite helpful. Take into consideration the dynamics of your work and social obligations. Make sure that you are reusing leftovers, as well. Purchase the supplies you need depending on the frequency of your cooking. You can make your purchases from the supermarket, online website, or even from the local farmer's market depending on how often you plan to cook. Also, depending on what you plan on cooking, use all the short-life ingredients within a couple of days or see to it that there is sufficient storage space in your refrigerator for the same, so they don't rot. Have a couple of basic ingredients and two or three ready-to-use sauces at home. This makes it easier to follow a diet. There are several paid and free mobile applications that will help you with planning in advance for your meals.

Always Make a Shopping List

Always make a shopping list before you go shopping. This will help you in buying only those ingredients that you actually need instead of picking up random ingredients. Make a list and stick to it. You can safely stay away from all sorts of junk if you do this. There are mobile applications you can make use of that will help you stay organized. If you are more old school, then a pen and paper will do the trick. Take into consideration the lists of Mediterranean diet-friendly foods that have been provided in this book.

Don't Buy Factory Farmed Fish

I
f you aren't able to get your hands on some fish caught in the wild, then it would be better to simply leave fish out of your diet. Avoid buying salmon and shrimp that has been farmed, as they may contain antibiotics and certain toxins. Fish that have been caught in the wild tend to have high levels of Omega-3 fatty acids and other proteins that are desirable. If wild-caught fish is too expensive, then avoid it. There are other protein sources for you to consider.

Be Careful When Purchasing Eggs or Chicken

Organic eggs are more expensive than the regular ones. The common labels that you will notice on eggs and chicken state free-range, pasture-raised, or organic. You need to understand the difference between all these labels so that you don't end up paying more for something just because it sounds fancy. You can purchase eggs and chicken from a local farmer, too. While buying chicken, you can buy the whole bird instead of a couple of cuts. This way, you can get all the cuts you want and the rest can be used to make chicken stock!

Avoid Convenience Foods

If you do your meal prep on weekends or whenever you are free, you don't have to spend unnecessarily on convenience foods. Buying pre-packed salad is more expensive than buying a head of lettuce. Don't take the easy way out. Don't buy trimmed green beans - just buy regular ones. It really doesn't take that long to get the job done. Stay away from all low-carb products. These products are not only expensive, but tend to contain all sorts of unhealthy ingredients as well. Always look at the list of ingredients before you buy something. If you don't understand something, then stay away from it.

Variety Matters

Make sure that you have included a variety of foods in your diet. No one likes to eat the same thing every single day. It gets boring and repetitive. Keep researching to find healthier alternatives. Apart from all the recipes given in this book, there are millions of healthy recipes that are available online that you can make use of. You can also share and trade recipes. Modify them to suit your needs and requirements. If the food starts to become boring, you will lose the motivation to continue.

Don't Starve

If you allow yourself to starve, then it will most certainly lead to an unnecessary binge. If your blood sugar levels are low, then you will automatically start craving carbs and sugary treats - the two things you must stay away from while following the Mediterranean diet. So, try to eat small meals throughout the day to keep hunger at bay.

Chapter Ten: Recipes for Wellness

After learning what meals to eat, it is now time to learn how to prepare them. This chapter contains a few useful recipes for anyone who wants to get into the Mediterranean diet. There is no need to go to a fancy restaurant to get a taste of these foods. The following recipes can easily be prepared in the comfort of your own home.

Breakfast Recipes: Starting the Day Right

Ditch your coffee and donut routine with one of the following breakfast meals straight out of the Mediterranean.

Orange-Banana Muffins
Ingredients:

- 3 cups of rolled oats

- ½ cup of almonds

- 1 tablespoon of baking powder

- 1 egg

- 1 cup of mandarin orange slices (drain and mash them with forks)

- 1 ripe banana, mashed

- ½ cup of brown sugar

- 1 tablespoon of vanilla

- 1 cup of unsweetened applesauce

- ½ cup of nonfat plain yogurt

- ½ cup of canned pumpkin puree

Steps:

1. Preheat your oven to 375 degrees

2. Combine oats and almonds using a blender to grind to flour. Pour this in a large mixing bowl and stir in some baking powder. Beat the egg in another bowl and add the oranges, banana, applesauce sugar and pumpkin.

3. Stir vanilla into the yogurt in a glass measure

4. Add 1/3 of the oat mixture to the banana mixture and stir until combined. Add half of the yogurt stirring until combined. Continue with the rest of the oats, yogurt and banana mixture.

5. Use non-stick cooking spray on 12 muffin cups before filling with batter. Bake for 20 minutes or until the middle sets. Remove from oven and cool for 15 minutes then remove from the muffin tin.

6. Cool completely before serving.

Almond Couscous

Ingredients:

- 1 cup of dry whole-grain couscous

- 2 cups of water

- ½ cup of currants

- ½ cup of coarsely chopped almonds

- 1 teaspoon each of ginger, cinnamon and cumin

- A dash each of salt, black pepper and red pepper

- 1 tablespoon of fruity olive oil

Steps:

1. Put the couscous in a bowl and add boiling water and cover immediately with a lid.

2. Let is stand for 5 minutes or until all the liquid is soaked up.

3. Stir almonds, spices and currants in and then olive oil after it is thoroughly combined. Let it stand at room temperature for 2 hours for the flavors to blend in.

4. Serve on the next day for the best-tasting breakfast.

Lunch Recipes: Midday Munching

Instead of burger, fries and a large soda, try one of these deliciously healthy lunch recipes the next time you eat your lunch.

Gazpacho

Ingredients:

- 4 pieces of seeded, chopped and peeled ripe tomatoes

- 2 cloves of minced garlic

- ½ cup of chopped bell pepper

- ½ cup of chopped and peeled cucumber

- ½ cup of chopped red onion

- ¼ cup of extra virgin olive oil

- ¼ teaspoon of ground cumin

- Juice of a freshly-squeezed lemon

- 1 cup of organic vegetable broth and enough ice cubes

- A dash of cayenne pepper

Steps:

1. Use a food processor with a metal blade to combine

all ingredients until smooth.

2. Chill mixture for at least 2 hours or overnight.

Enough for 4 servings

Macedonian Salad
Ingredients:

- 1 piece of lemon at room temperature

- 1 cup of seedless grapes

- 1 cup of halved strawberries

- 1 cup of melon cubes or balls

- 1 cup of cubed peaches

- ½ cup of red wine

- ¼ cup of sugar

Steps:

1. Roll the lemon on the counter and cut into quarters then set aside.

2. Combine remaining fruits in a large bowl and squeeze the lemon quarters over them. Stir gently and avoid the fruit from breaking or getting mashed.

3. Sprinkle with a little sugar and drizzle with wine then

toss gently.

4. Let it stand at room temperature for 10 to 15 minutes then serve.

Chicken España
Ingredients:

- 1 cut-up chicken

- 3 cloves of minced garlic

- 2 tablespoons of chopped fresh parsley

- 1 tablespoon of dried oregano leaves

- ½ cup of pitted ripe olives

- ¼ cup of extra virgin olive oil

- ¼ cup of dry white wine

- ¼ cup of packed brown sugar

- ¼ cup of red wine vinegar

Steps:

1. Mix in vinegar, oil, olives, garlic and oregano. Pour this mixture on the chicken in a Ziplock bag.

2. Let the chicken marinade in the refrigerator for 2 hours with occasional turning.

3. Put the chicken in a shallow baking dish and sprinkle with brown sugar.

4. Pour wine into the pan and cook at 350 degrees for an hour or until thoroughly cooked with basting every 20 minutes.

5. Sprinkle parsley before serving.

Makes 4 to 6 servings

Herb-Roasted Mediterranean Vegetables
Ingredients:

- 8 cups of assorted vegetables

- 2 cloves of minced garlic

- 2 teaspoons of dried rosemary leaves

- 1 teaspoon of salt

- ½ cup of shredded Parmesan cheese

- ¼ cup of extra virgin olive oil

Steps:

1. Toss the vegetables together with garlic, oil, salt and rosemary and place in a large shallow pan.

2. Bake at 375 degrees in the oven for 40 minutes or until the vegetables become tender. Stir once or twice

during cooking.

3. Sprinkle the cheese if desired.

Makes 6 to 8 servings

Spicy Vegetable Couscous
Ingredients:

- 1 cup of couscous

- 1 cup of chopped zucchini and red onion

- ½ cup of grated carrots

- 1 can of chicken broth

- 1 can of rinsed and drained garbanzo beans

- 1 clove of minced garlic

- 2 tablespoons of extra virgin olive oil

- ½ teaspoon each of ground cumin, salt, curry powder and red pepper flakes

Steps:

1. Bring broth to a boil and stir in couscous. Remove this from the heat.

2. Let it stand covered for 5 minutes then heat in a large skillet.

3. Add in the zucchini, carrots, onion and garlic cooking for 5 minutes or until it becomes tender with occasional stirring.

4. Add in the seasonings, beans and couscous and cook until heated thoroughly for 2 minutes.

Makes 6 servings

Falafel with Tomato–Cucumber Relish
Ingredients:

- 15-ounce can of rinsed and drained garbanzo beans

- 2 cloves of minced garlic

- 1 coarsely-chopped medium-sized onion

- 1 large lightly beaten egg

- 1 cup of dry whole-wheat bread crumbs

- 1 tablespoon of fresh lemon juice

- 1 teaspoon of dried oregano

- ½ teaspoon of ground cumin

- Olive oil cooking spray

- Tomato-Cucumber relish

- Freshly-ground black pepper and salt to taste

Steps:

1. Process the garbanzo beans, parsley, garlic, onion, cumin and oregano in a food processor fitted with a metal blade.

2. Season with lemon juice, pepper and salt and stir in the bread crumbs and egg

3. Spread other bread crumbs on a plate. Use your hands to form 16 round balls out of the bean mixture and roll them on the bread crumbs for coating. Set these balls on wax paper.

4. Spray a large skillet with your cooking spray and use medium heat until hot. Add falafel balls to cook until browned for about 10 minutes.

5. Serve with Tomato-Cucumber relish or fresh greens and pita halves.

Makes 4 servings

Tomato-Cucumber Relish
Ingredients:

- ½ cup of chopped cucumber

- ½ cup of chopped tomato

- 1/3 cup of nonfat plain yogurt

- ¼ teaspoon of dried mint

- Freshly-ground black pepper and salt to taste

Steps:

1. Combine all ingredients in a small bowl.

2. Season with salt and pepper to taste

Makes 4 servings

Snacks: Taking A Break from It All

Junk foods are not the only things you can reach out to during your break time. For a healthier snack time, try one of the following recipes yourself.

Olive Oil Cheese Crisps

Ingredients:

- 6 slices of whole-grain bread of your choice

- 3 cloves of peeled and halved garlic

- ¼ cup of extra virgin olive oil

- ¼ cup of grated Parmesan cheese

- A dash of sea salt

Steps:

1. Cut the slices of bread into strips around an inch

wide. Brush these strips with olive oil on both sides and spread them on a cooking sheet.

2. Broil strips until crispy and golden brown. Remove the strips and brush the sides with garlic cloves.

3. Sprinkle with cheese and season with sea salt. Return these to the broiler and cook until cheese melts.

4. Remove from broiler and cool down before serving. Serve with dip or by itself.

Makes 6 servings

Caponata
Ingredients:

- 1 medium eggplant

- 1 chopped medium red bell pepper

- 1 chopped medium yellow bell pepper

- 1 tablespoon of sea salt

- 1 tablespoon of red wine vinegar

- 1 tablespoon of chopped fresh basil

- 1 tablespoon of chopped fresh Italian parsley

- 1 cup of pitted and coarsely chopped black olives

- ½ teaspoon of red pepper flakes

- ¼ cup of rinsed and drained capers

- 2 teaspoons of sugar

- 2 cloves of minced garlic

- 6 pieces of blanched and peeled tomatoes or 1 large can of tomatoes

Steps:

1. Cut the eggplant into cubes and put in colander and toss with sea salt. Place a paper towel over this and put colander on the sink. Top with a plate to weigh down the eggplant. Allow for 30 minutes to drain.

2. Spray olive oil cooking spray on skillet and heat over medium-high fire. Rinse and dry eggplant and cook in skillet.

3. Lower fire to medium-low and add onion, garlic and olive oil. Sauté for about 15 minutes until onion is soft.

4. Add tomatoes, bell peppers, red pepper flakes, sugar and vinegar and cook until the mixture thickens for about 30 minutes. Continue simmering for another 30 minutes.

5. Add olives, parsley, basil and capers and stir

thoroughly. Remove caponata from heat and let it stand to cool down.

6. Serve right away or store in an airtight container.

Makes 6 servings

Broiled Tomatoes
Ingredients:

- ½ teaspoon of sea salt

- ¼ cup of hard and dry bread crumbs

- 2 tablespoons of chopped fresh basil or 2 teaspoons of dried basils

- 2 tablespoons of grated Parmesan cheese

- 2 tablespoons of extra virgin olive oil

- 6 pieces of medium fresh tomatoes

Steps:

1. Core tomatoes and cut them in half going through the middle.

2. Heat the olive oil in a skillet over a medium-high fire until the aroma is released for about 5 minutes.

3. Put the tomatoes with the cut side down and cook until crispy for another 5 minutes. Scoop them up

with a spatula and add a sprinkle of salt, cheese, basil and bread crumbs.

4. Broil tomatoes on a broiler pan until the cheese melts and the tomato is a crispy golden brown.

Makes 6 servings

Dinner: Ending the Day Right

Nothing beats a healthy, home-cooked meal after coming home from work. The following recipes make sure that you always come home to a healthy meal after a long day at the office.

Swordfish Steaks with Tomato-Caper Sauce
Ingredients:

- 4 pieces of grilled or broiled swordfish steaks around 6 ounces each

- 2 pieces of large seeded and chopped tomatoes

- 1 clove of minced garlic

- 1 teaspoon of dried tarragon

- 1 teaspoon of extra virgin olive oil

- ¼ cup of capers

- Black pepper and sea salt to taste

Steps:

1. Combine the capers, tarragon, garlic, pepper, salt, oil and tomatoes.

2. Serve at room temperature over the swordfish steaks or other kind of white meat.

Makes 4 servings

Greek Salad

Ingredients:

- 10 pieces of pitted kalamata or other Greek olives of high quality

- 2 cups of bite-sized Romaine lettuce pieces

- 2 pieces of medium tomatoes cut into wedges

- 1 tablespoon of minced fresh Italian parsley

- ½ cup of red onions sliced thinly

- ½ cup of cucumbers sliced thinly

- ½ cup of green bell peppers sliced thinly

- ½ cup of red bell peppers sliced thinly

- ½ cup of crumbled feta cheese of good quality

(Dressing)

- 1 small clove of minced garlic

- 1 tablespoon of fresh lemon juice

- ½ teaspoon of minced fresh oregano

- ¼ cup of extra virgin olive oil

Steps:

1. Spread Romaine lettuce on a platter and arrange tomato wedges over them.

2. Combine the onions, peppers, parsley, half of the feta cheese and cucumbers in a bowl. Spread this over the tomato and lettuce and top with olives and the rest of the feta cheese.

3. Whisk the oil, lemon juice, garlic and oregano together to make the dressing. Drizzle this over the salad and toss before serving.

4. Makes 4 servings

Olive Oil Vinaigrette

Ingredients:

- 2 tablespoons of balsamic vinegar, red wine vinegar of good quality or fresh lemon juice

- 1 clove of minced garlic

- 1 teaspoon of salt

- ½ cup of extra virgin olive oil

- A dash of freshly-ground black pepper

Steps:

1. Combine vinegar or lemon juice, salt, garlic and pepper in a small bowl.

2. Whisk the olive oil in until it is well-blended and serve right away over your salad of choice.

Makes 8 tablespoons of salad dressing enough for 4 to 6 people

Mediterranean Citrus Chicken
Ingredients:

- 4 pieces of boneless chicken breast halves of 4 ounce each

- 2 cups of fresh greens

- 1 teaspoon of olive oil

- 1 teaspoon of cornstarch

- 1 teaspoon of water

- 1 tablespoon of honey

- ¼ cup of chicken broth

- Juice and zest from one of the following:

- 1 large orange

- 1 large lemon

- 1 large lime

- 1 small grapefruit

- 1 piece of lime with the ends cut off (for garnish)

- Sprigs of Italian parsley (for garnish)

Steps:

1. Combine all citrus juices in a measuring cup and the zests in a small bowl. Place a plastic bag in a small tray and pour half of the juice in.

2. Add the chicken and sprinkle half the zest. Seal the bag and lay it on the baking pan. Turn it over several times making sure that the chicken is covered well.

3. Place this on the refrigerator and marinade for at least 2 hours or overnight. Store the rest of the zest and juice in an airtight bowl.

4. Put chicken broth and olive oil in a non-stick skillet with a medium-high fire until it simmers. Add the chicken without the marinade and reduce heat to

medium.

5. Cook the chicken until the pink disappears for about 20 to 25 minutes. Do not forget to turn halfway.

6. Combine the reserved zest and juice in a separate saucepan over a medium-low fire for 5 minutes. Make paste with the cornstarch and water. Whisk this with the juice mixture and stir constantly until the mixture thickens for about 15 minutes and remove from heat.

7. Cover your platter with fresh greens and place the chicken over these. Drizzle with a bit of sauce and add in the rest of the zest. Arrange the slices of lime and parsley sprigs for garnish.

Makes 4 servings

Conclusion

The healthier lifestyle in the Mediterranean proves one very important thing. Clearly, living and eating healthy is a choice anyone can make regardless of your current situation.

It is all a matter of taking the initiative to make the necessary changes to live healthy. With increased vitality, less risk from chronic diseases and a longer life, who would not want to?

This eBook has presented everything you need to know to become a healthier person through the Mediterranean diet. Now go out there and start applying everything you have learned here.

References:

MUFA-rich foods may help reduce your risk for heart disease. (2019). Retrieved from https://www.mayoclinic.org/healthy-lifestyle/nutrition-and-healthy-eating/expert-answers/mufas/faq-20057775

5 Mediterranean Diet Myths...Busted! | Nutrition By Carrie. (2019). Retrieved from https://www.nutritionbycarrie.com/2017/09/mediterranean-diet-myths.html

10 Simple Ways to Follow the Mediterranean Diet. (2019). Retrieved from https://www.betternutrition.com/features-dept/mediterranean-diet

Mediterranean Diet Mistakes You're Probably Making | Bottom Line Inc. (2019). Retrieved from https://bottomlineinc.com/health/diet-nutrition/mediterranean-diet-mistakes-youre-probably-making

17 Arse-kicking Strategies to Stick to Your Diet and Get Fit : zen habits. (2019). Retrieved from https://zenhabits.net/17-arse-kicking-strategies-to-stick-to-your-diet-and-get-fit/

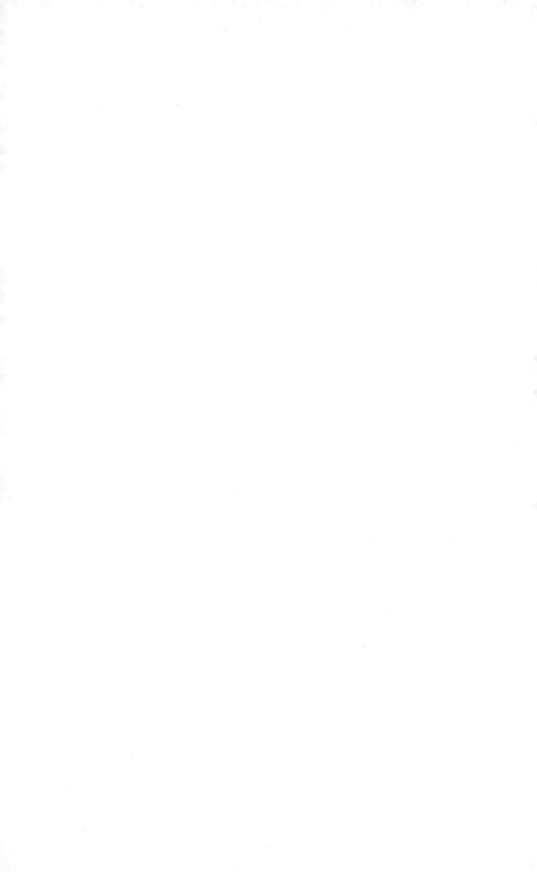

PART II - Fat Loss

For Women And Men

Medical Advisory

The information and workout procedures provided in this guide are very intense and should not be attempted by anyone unless a doctor has cleared you for such an intense workout.

If you have any existing health problems that would prohibit you from taking part in any of these activities, you should refrain.

As always, you should clear this program with your doctor before you begin.

SERIOUSLY – THIS IS AN EXTREME PROGRAM. IT IS NOT FOR EVERYONE. THOSE WITH PRE-EXISTING MEDICAL CONDITIONS SHOULD NOT ATTEMPT THIS PROGRAM. NO ONE SHOULD ATTEMPT THIS PROGRAM WITHOUT PRIOR CLEARANCE FROM YOUR DOCTOR.

A Cheat Code For Getting Lean?

Up up, down down, left right, left right, b, a, select start. If you're a child of the 80's, you'll recognize the sequence above as the famous "cheat code" for the video game, Contra.

You'd just tap that sequence in on the start screen and boom – unlimited lives. It was the ultimate "cheat code."

In some ways, this manual is nothing more than a cheat code. A cheat code for getting lean as fast as possible.

Inside these pages you'll discover a method of weight loss that works so fast, it will feel like cheating. To be clear, this is not about doing anything illegal. Obviously, some people go the route of using illegal or prescription drugs or even undergoing surgery to lose weight.

Whether you consider those methods cheating or not, that is NOT what this book is all about.

But as the saying goes, "All is fair in love and war" and make no mistake about it – an attempt to get lean is an all-out war on your stored body fat.

So you owe it to yourself to know "every trick in the book" before you step on the battlefield. You can decide for yourself which tricks you choose to employ, and which tricks are best left untouched.

Keep in mind, most of the fat loss tricks I'm going to be sharing with you are OPTIONAL. For example, later in this book I'll be showing you a way you can actually use alcoholic drinks to speed UP fat loss.

Does this mean you MUST drink booze in order to lose weight? Or course not. That would be silly. Obviously, you can lose fat quickly without drinking alcohol. However, I'm including the tip because I know a lot of people have been told you must swear off alcohol if you want to get lean. In this book, I'll show you why that's not true. But remember, the decision to use alcohol is yours and yours alone and it is again, 100% optional.

I'll give you a number of tips that will be labeled "optional." You can use them if you want to speed things up or make the process easier, but when it comes to getting lean quickly the "secret" always has been and always will be getting just a few things right. Let's dive in...

How To Lose 9 Pounds Of Fat In 3 Days

I want to shatter a long-standing myth about fat loss right out of the gate. In the rest of this book, I'll disprove a number of myths about fat loss.

So we may as well kill this myth right off the bat. You've not doubt heard that the best you can hope for is losing two pounds of fat in a week. Somewhere along the line that benchmark became accepted as gospel. But published, peer-reviewed research PROVES that's a myth.

In fact there's actually a way you can lose 8.36 pounds of fat in the next 72 hours. Check it out:

Researchers conducted a study called "A time-efficient reduction of fat mass in 4 days with exercise and caloric restriction."

And the methodology was really quite simple.

Researchers took overweight individuals and put them on what was essentially a starvation diet --- only 300 calories per day for 4 days. Then they had the individuals walk at a slow pace (roughly 2.7 mph) for 8 hours a day!

The results were astonishing. The average person lost 3.8kg of pure body fat – that's 8.36 pounds of fat.

Now, it's worth mentioning that the subjects also lost lean mass as well. But before you freak out, keep in mind that the subjects regained the lean mass after the 4 day diet experiment was over. This shows us that the lean mass lost was most likely water and glycogen, not actual muscle tissue.

But there's a couple more interesting aspects of this study… #1) Even after the day experiment was over and the subjects resumed normal eating and stopped walking for 8 hours a day, they continued to lose fat.

And…

#2) When compared with other dieters a year later… the group that took part in the 4-day experiment were MORE successful at keeping the weight off even a full year after the experiment was over.

This sounds completely counter-intuitive especially if you believe the lie that crash diets are bad because you will automatically regain all the weight.

To shed some light on why dieters were more successful a year after the crash diet, look at it like this: If you had a goal to save up $25,000 in cash, how much more motivated would you be to achieve your goal if a long-lost uncle suddenly gifted you $15,000?

Suddenly, the idea of saving $25,000 in cash is much more manageable because your uncle has essentially given you a "running start.'

This 4-day crash diet with extreme exercise does the same thing: It gives you a massive "running start" towards achieving your goal. Most people want to lose between 10 - 20 pounds of fat. Which could take anywhere from 12 weeks to 12 months for the average person.

But if you can drop 8 pounds of pure fat in the first 4 days, then you can hit your goal much faster and spend less time dieting and more time maintaining.

So if you're up for the challenge, here's how to set up your own fat loss kick-start. By the way, this is OPTIONAL. You do not need to attempt this to hit your goal, it is only for people who want to hit the ground running and lose a bunch of fat in their first week on the program.

First even though the original research used a 4-day plan, I recommend just a 3-day kick start. This is simply because this plan is extremely tough and 3 days is enough for our purposes.

Remember, we're only using this to kick -start weight loss and immediately following this plan you will jump into the rest of the program from this manual.

Second, I don't think most people will be able to walk 8 hours a day. If you can, great. But if you're like me and have a desk job and you can't just walk around all day, that's ok.

Just try to be as active as you can and you'll still lose plenty of fat on this plan.

Third: You'll want to consume roughly 300 calories per day on this plan. And you want mostly protein.

Here is what I ate on this plan:

Carb Control Shakes

You can find these or something similar in most grocery stores now day.

They are typically sold in packs of 4.

Pre-cooked Southwest Chicken Strips: 200 calories.

Pretty sure these are designed to be used on salads, but I would
just heat them up for a minute in the microwave and eat them plain.

Yes, that's not very much food and that's exactly why this plan is only 3 days long.

There is no way of predicting how much fat you'll lose during these 3 days as much of it will depend on how much walking you are able to do.

When I did this 3 day experiment I lost over 6 pounds without doing much walking (I have a desk job so I tried to walk in the morning before work, for a few minutes on my lunch break and for a few minutes at night but I definitely didn't walk for 8 hours a day.)

Make no mistake, this is an OPTIONAL kick start plan. But if you choose to try this, not only will you lose a bunch of fat in the first 3 days, you'll also end up shrinking your stomach so that your feelings of hunger will be greatly reduced beginning on day 4.

If you think this is too extreme, don't worry about it and just skip it. We'll over the regular diet plan beginning in the next chapter.

The regular diet plan also seem a bit extreme but those that do the 3-day kickstart first will find that an ordinary diet suddenly becomes much easier.

About This Manual

This is not a book of theory or hypothesis. This a field-guide. An "in-the trenches" overview of real world experience on what I believe is the fastest and easiest way to get lean and stay lean.

Much of what I'm about to show you will fly in the face of what your average personal trainer or dietician believes to be true. If that bothers you, than this program isn't right for you.

I have included only a few scientific references in this program. Because this isn't a manual for pondering the latest scientific developments in the worlds of diet and exercise science. This is a book for getting and staying ultra-lean.

The method works – no matter what science or other (flabby) personal trainers say. If you're skeptical, try the first 13 days and you'll become a believer.

Lastly, a note for women. Very few women will ever read this book. And if any women are reading this, very few will ever attempt the program. If you are a woman, there's no reason you can't follow this program. I've included the necessary adjustments to make where applicable.

Why Get Lean

Yeah, I know. This chapter might sound odd. After all, if you're reading this book we can all assume you already know why you want to get lean. But I want to lay some more evidence on you. Keep this stuff in mind when your willpower gets weak.

Note To Women: The following section is mostly for men. There are host of female specific physiological and psychological advantages to getting lean. You'll feel better, you'll look better, clothes fit better, etc... the list goes on.

MEN: If you've got high levels of body fat, your body is an estrogen factory. Your excess fat cells create higher than normal estrogen levels, which makes every calorie you eat far more likely to be stored as fat. Which creates a vicious cycle, killing your testosterone levels and killing your motivation to ever achieve anything.

In short, carrying excess body fat turns men in to women. So the single greatest benefit just might be the fact that getting leaner turns your body into a testosterone-fueled machine.

If you are lean and you over-eat, your body will shift a greater percentage of those calories towards muscle. If you are overweight and you over-eat, a greater percentage gets shifted to fat.

Sounds unfair? It is unfair. Cry about it. Or just sack up and make the decision to get ultra-lean.

Lean men LOOK bigger. It's true. When your muscles aren't covered in fat, you look bigger and more muscular than you really are.

Abs? The best way to getting better abs is to lose body fat. Once you're down to single digit levels of body fat, your abs will be popping out like never before.

Do It Because Most Can't: Here's the simple truth about why getting lean is so awesome:

Most people can't do it. You can't buy this. You can't bargain for this. You can't trade for this. Getting lean can only be EARNED.

Wealth can be transferred. Riches can be stolen. Good looks can come from your parents or be purchased at the plastic surgeon. But getting a lean & ripped physique can only be earned.

People recognize this and you'll feel the instant respect (and often pure hatred – more on this later) coming from others once they see your level of leanness.

Congrats! You're Fatter Than You Think

Time to figure out how fat you actually are. AKA – your starting point. Unfortunately, people frequently get this wrong. It's a running joke that whenever someone says they are "about 10% body fat" you can pretty much guarantee they're closer to 15%. If they say they are 15% they are probably closer to 22%. And so on...

So how fat are you really? The only way to know for sure is to go out and get a DEXA scan. Search on Internet "Dexa body fat scan" in your area to see if there's any nearby facility close to you that does these scans.

If you can get one of these done, I highly recommend it as it's the only way to know for sure exactly how much fat you're carrying.

If you live near a major city you should be able to find an establishment that offers once of these scans. However, here's an alternative:

I've got a free and simple body fat calculator on my blog. It's actually pretty accurate for most people. In fact, this calculator routinely estimates my body fat within 1% of what my DEXA scan reads.

Ok, so now you know you're starting point. You've gotten a DEXA scan or you've used the body fat calculator above.

Either way, you're already trying to invent some type of rationalization as to why these figures are wrong and why you're actually leaner than what the numbers say.

Stop. Just stop. Yes, you're fatter than you thought. Get over it.

Because your starting point doesn't really matter. The goal is getting lean. And if you follow this program, you'll get there sooner than you thought possible.

100% Mental

Make no mistake about it. Getting and staying ultra-lean is 100% mental. I am going to show you the exact system to follow to achieve a lean physique in a matter of weeks.

There is literally nothing you need to figure out on your own. All you need to do is follow the instructions as written. The program itself is very simple and straightforward. If you actually follow the instructions, you cannot fail.

If you fail, you simply did not follow the instructions. You can make any excuse you want, but the truth of the matter is this: If you fail, you are mentally weak.

There is no other alternative. There will be days when you don't want to stick with the program. There will be days when you look in the mirror and wonder if it's actually working.

And there will be moments when you'll be tempted to abandon your goals and join the ranks of the obese cows around you mashing cake into their faces at every opportunity. ("But it's ma third-cousins nephew's 57th birthday party. I had to!")

If you fail, you are mentally weak.

This program is difficult, but not impossible. And best of all, it's fast. You'll lose more fat on this diet in 6 weeks than most people do in 6 months. But if you can't handle being on a diet for 6 weeks, then it's not because your life is too busy or your "body is different", it's because you are mentally weak.

Only the mentally strong can achieve a lean physique. So before you even go to the next page, know that your success or failure on this program will rest on the strength of your mind.

Most people aren't mentally strong enough to achieve a lean & fit physique. Just as most people aren't mentally strong enough to quit smoking, learn a new skill, change careers, or better themselves in any way.

With belaboring this point too much, the key to getting lean fast is dealing with hunger. And 90% of hunger is actually in your mind. So if you're not mentally strong enough to deal with hunger (fake hunger, not actual hunger – more on this later), you will fail.

I'm reminded of the age-old marshmallow experiment. You've heard the story. Scientists put a bunch of toddlers in a room and told them they could have 1 marshmallow now. Or if they could wait, they could have 2 marshmallows later.

Most kids weren't able to wait and immediately scarfed down their single marshmallow. Scientists followed up with those that were able to delay gratification in exchange for two marshmallows and found that the kids who successfully waited for 2 marshmallows were more successful in life in general.

To succeed with this method (or to succeed with anything in life), you need to master the art of delaying gratification. You will be allowed to eat every junk food your heart desires...and in copious quantities as well. But not always right when you want it.

That's the essence of mental strength: The art of delaying gratification. Most people cannot do this.

If you're reading this, chances are you're better than most people. Mentally stronger, at least. But we'll find out.

Normal Diet Vs Bodybuilding/Fitness Diets Vs This Method

For regular people, counting calories is a huge stumbling block. Diet authors know that regular people simply won't count calories.

So they invent diets that work to restrict calories without making dieters actually count anything.

This chart sums that up perfectly.

How Named Diets Work for Weight Loss

Diet Name	Short Description	How it Works
Low Carb	Eat fewer carbs and more foods rich in protein and fats	By creating a caloric deficit
Ketogenic	Eat almost no carbs, some protein and mostly fats	By creating a caloric deficit
Low Fat	Avoid foods high in fats and eat mostly protein and carbs	By creating a caloric deficit
Intermittent Fasting	Restrict your eating period to only a few hours every day	By creating a caloric deficit
Weight Watchers	Points based system to help with portion control	By creating a caloric deficit
Paleo	Eat only minimally-processed "paleolithic" foods	By creating a caloric deficit

Atkins figured out that if you told people they could lose weight by cutting out all carbs, they could lose weight without counting calories.

Of course, it only works for about 2 weeks. I'm not even joking. Over a 6 month period, most diets see all their success in the first 2 weeks, and then flounder for the next 24 weeks.

Bodybuilding or fitness-based diets are a little bit better. Because people interested in bodybuilding or fitness routines are usually willing to apply a little more effort to achieve their goals and so calorie-counting is acceptable.

But the diets themselves are still stupid. You'll often read recommendations to "keep your protein at 1 gram per pound of bodyweight per day" or "eat 2,000 calories per and do 30 minutes of cardio" every night.

And that's the single biggest flaw with even the more "advanced" bodybuilding diets. They set the initial calorie intake way to high and then ask you to do hours of cardio to account for the mistake.

Even if you follow their diet successfully, the traditional bodybuilding/fitness diet is dreadfully slow. Most bodybuilding and fitness competitors will diet for 12-16 weeks before a competition, eschewing all sense of normality or a real life.

They'll suffer for 3-4 months to end up getting in stage-ready condition for 1 day. Then they'll binge afterward and do it all again a few weeks later.

This method is different. What takes most people 12-16 weeks we'll accomplish in half the time. And then I'll show you how to easily maintain your newfound level of leanness with less effort than you ever thought possible.

It's a smarter way to diet. And it all begins on the next page...

The Firs Week

Ok, time to dive into the nuts & bolts of the actual diet plan. We're going map this out in phases. In this chapter, I'll cover the first week of the diet.

The first week is the hardest. Honestly, just the first few days really. They aren't brutally difficult, but they are more difficult than most diets.

If you can handle the first few days, then congrats – you can handle the rest of the diet and it will only be a matter of time until you reach your goal.

The Problem With Most Diets

As I hinted at earlier, the problem with most diets is that they set your caloric intake levels too high, and then force you to do an hour (or more) of cardio per day in the hopes of creating a reasonable caloric deficit.

This causes people to fail for 3 reasons:

#1) Studies show that people vastly UNDERestimate how many calories they are truly consuming.

#2) Studies also show that people vastly OVERestimate how many calories they are truly burning from exercise.
#3) Lastly, it's extremely difficult to stay on a diet if you're not seeing results.

So here's how this usually plays out. Your average guy with an office job and who exercises or plays sports a few times a week needs roughly 2,500 calories per day to maintain his bodyweight.

He decides he wants to lose some weight so he talks to a registered dietician (ha! First mistake) and she tells him to simply eat less and move more. She recommends he aims for a 500 calorie-deficit from diet and that he adds some additional cardio sessions to his week.

Then she charges him $85 for the 15 minute conversation and saunters away. So now our poor chap is supposed to eat 2,000 calories per day, do a bit more cardio throughout the week and hopefully achieve his goals.

What happens?

Well, he loses some water weight during the first week simply by making cleaner food choices. The next week he only loses a pound. During week 3 he doesn't lose a single pound and his motivation falls through the floor. He grits his teeth and sticks with it for another week, only to not lose a single pound in week 4.

He quits, rewards himself with a cheat day and moves on to the next diet plan.

This cycle continues over and over for the next 12 months. A year of his life goes down the drain and he ends up exactly the same (or even more likely – fatter) than he was when he started out.

As I mentioned, you, me, heck humans in general – we're all pretty awful at estimating how many calories we're eating. So if we set out to eat 2,000 calories, there's a good chance we're probably eating 2,300 or even 2,500 calories a day.

And we're just as bad at estimating how many calories we're burning from exercise. So if we set out to burn 500 calories, there's a good chance we're really only burning 100 or 175 calories.

When you combine those factors, a guy who attempts to eat 2,000 calories and burn 500 calories a day via exercise will actually be eating 2,300 calories and burning only 175 calories per day via exercise.

Which means IF he loses any fat, he's only going to lose a tiny amount of fat – not even enough to show the results in the mirror or on the scale.

So he'll lose motivation and quit.

The Underground Fat Loss Method Is Different

We're not going to mess around. We're going to set calories as low as possible right from the jump to ENSURE that we're hacking off as much body fat as we can on a daily basis.

We're not even going to bother with cardio – if you want to do some fine – but we're not going to try and calculate how many calories cardio burns.

We're going to use resistance-training as a tool to maintain and build lean muscle – not to burn calories.

We'll use calculated "cheats" for mental sanity and to restore hormone levels and muscle fullness. And we'll use a large daily caloric deficit to incinerate body fat so that you see results almost on a day-by-day basis.

The end result? We're going to accomplish in 4-6 weeks what takes most dieter 16 weeks to 6 months to accomplish.

How Many Calories?

For most people, the daily calorie target will be 1,250 calories. This is the standard recommendation for average-sized males with desk jobs and a few hours of exercise or sport- related activities per week.

Women – or very small men – (under 140lbs) will want to aim for 1,000 calories per day.

Larger men (over 250lbs) or men with manual labor jobs will want to shoot for 1,500 calories per day.

Right now you're probably thinking "that's not very many calories" and you are correct – it's not. And that's exactly the point.

By supplying only a minimum level of calories, your body is forced to make up the difference by burning calories you have stored in your body – body fat.

A lot of people get tripped up on the idea that not eating enough calories is somehow a problem when trying to lose weight.
You wouldn't believe how many people come to me and say they can't seem to lose any weight and they suspect the reason is because they aren't eating enough.

Yeah, right.

That's like saying "I can't seem to save any money... and I suspect it's because I'm not spending enough!"

It makes no sense. Most guys believe if you don't eat enough calories your muscle will waste away. Most women believe if you don't eat enough calories it will jack up your hormones or "damage your metabolism."

Bullshit. People cling to these myths and lies because deep down they want to believe the magical idea that you can somehow burn more fat by eating more. If that idea worked, you wouldn't be reading this book.

The uncomfortable truth is this – you need to eat LESS— probably far less than you thought – to actually lose fat at a meaningful pace.

Sure, in theory you can lose weight by just cutting your calories by 100 or 200 per day. But in reality, unless you create a SIGNIFICANT daily caloric deficit, you'll never get lean.

So instead of wondering if the calories are "too low" just trust me on this and follow this diet for the first week.

Why A Week?

As I already mentioned, the first few days will be toughest. If you can "win" the first few days, you're golden. The diet doesn't change that much after the first few days, but your stomach will shrink and your hunger levels drop dramatically.

Which means you might find yourself starving around the clock on day 2, but by day 4 you'll find that you're really not all that hungry.

How Often To Eat?

It doesn't matter. The idea that 6 meals a day is better than 3, or that 3 meals a day is better than 2 is complete nonsense.

Eat 6 meals a day or eat 1 meal a day, it doesn't matter – as long as you hit your calorie targets, the number of meals makes no difference.

Having said that, because of the low number of calories on this plan, most people will do better with 1 or 2 meals a day.

Again, you COULD eat 6 meals if you want, but that means each meal has to be about 200 calories and that's just kind of a pain in the ass to deal with.

What To Eat?

Now we come to the million-dollar question. People always think there are some magical foods or some forbidden foods when it comes to losing fat.

But the truth is, as long as you stay under your calorie requirements for the day, the choice of foods doesn't really matter.

The caveat of course if that if you eat cake and cookies you will not get full and you'll hit your calorie limit after just a few bites. But if you choose whole foods, you'll be able to eat a lot more food and you'll feel better.

To that end, there are some foods that I feel are a bit "magical" in that they provide a high level of fullness/satiety without a massive calorie hit. The full list is in a later chapter.

I'll also show you a few sample days from my own eating plan so you can get a feel for what foods I choose when trying to eat 1,250 calories a day.

Macro-Nutrients?

Listen – I really don't care about macronutrients. I know, I know. Most people are obsessed with getting their "macros" right.

Honestly, it doesn't matter. Some days I eat high fat and low carb. Some days I eat high carb and low fat. Some days I eat pizza. (Pizza is high carb AND high fat, so it's not an ideal meal for losing fat.) However, as long as you stay under your calorie target you will still lose fat. So yes, you can eat pizza and still lose fat.

But here is a tip:

When you're trying to eat a lower number of calories, if you can restrict a certain macronutrient, you can eat a lot more food (and increase fullness.)

For example, if you eat a meal that's high in carbohydrates and high in protein, but very low in fat you'll be able to consume way more food (while still staying under your caloric target) than if you try and hit your caloric targets with a more "balanced" approach.

So if you feel like eating a low-carb diet for a couple days, and then switching to a higher carb diet for a day, have at it. Don't stress about macros. Stay under your calorie targets consistently and you'll lose fat no matter what macros you are eating.

Cheat days (more on this later) will be lower-protein days. So over the course of a week, you'll have some low carb days, some low fat days and perhaps one low protein day.

Which means you'll never get "too low" on any given macronutrient.

This method allows you to avoid the crappy feeling that comes from following a low-carb diet for an extended period, avoid the negative effects of following a low-fat diet for an extended period of time and most days keep your protein intake a little bit higher with is good for fullness and muscle recovery.

Want a cookie? Fine, have it. But add to the MyFitnessPal app and see how many calories it takes up. You might for yourself opting for celery instead.

Pizza night with the family? Go right ahead. But make sure you are counting calories with the MyFitnessPal app and only eat enough to stay under your limit for the day.

It really is that simple. And that's why I've isolated the first few days. Because whatever questions you THINK you may have about this plan are usually resolved by diving in and STARTING the plan for a few days.

So if your head is swimming with questions right now, I'd encourage you to A) finish the book and B) commit to starting the plan for at least the first few days.

After a few days of experience, you'll find the plan of attack is now much clearer. Let's move on...

The Firs Two Weeks

Don't make any changes for the first two weeks. You're going to continue with the same daily calorie target of 1,250 (for most people) every day. You're going to lose weight at a very quick pace.

Hunger pangs will have mostly subsided after the first few days and now you've probably fallen into a groove.

You've probably found a few food items that work well for you, and for the most part you'll eat these food items on a fairly regular basis. (Again, the list of foods revealed later in this manual will help with this.)

Most people will end up losing 5-10 pounds in these first two weeks. Some people will lose more. Much of this is water weight, but it's also fat as well because we're using an extreme caloric deficit.

After 13 consecutive days eating in this fashion, you'll have finally earned your first cheat/refeed day. We'll cover the rules for the cheat/refeed day in the next chapter.

Day 14: The Cheat/Refeed Day

Traditional diets have you running a very minor caloric deficit for 6 days and then reward that insanely low level of commitment with a full-day free-for-all binge session that often wipes out any progress made during the initial six days of dieting.

The Underground Fat Loss Method will be different. First, we're using a far more extreme caloric deficit.
Second rather than scheduling a cheat meal every week, we're pushing it to every 14th day (at least during the first month of this program.)

Third: Our cheat/refeed days are not going to be no-hold barred free for all, but rather a calculated approach to restore glycogen levels, muscle fullness and hormone levels.

4th and finally, we're going to implement a very strict pre- and POST cheat day strategy to minimize the carry-over effect.

So here is the cheat/refeed strategy:

1. You must fast all day on the day of your cheat/refeed day.
2. Confine your cheat/refeed calories to a 4 hour window. On normal days, I don't care if you eat 6 small meals per day. But on your cheat/refeed day, I want you to confine all calories to a single big feast.

   This way we're giving the body one big 'hit' of insulin and allowing the body to immediately start to process the calories and insulin spike, rather than spacing it out over time.
3. Keep cheat day calories at 2,500 – 3,000 calories total. Most people don't realize this but if you give yourself a full "cheat day" you can easily consume 6,000, 8,000 calories or more which would completely undo a week of dieting. But by capping your calories on your cheat/refeed meal at 2,500 – 3,000 you are giving your body a small surplus to

restore hormone levels, without undoing too much of your prior work. So again, use the MyFitnessPal app or something similar to track calories on your cheat day.

4. Eat whatever you want for your cheat/refeed meals. Junk food is fine. High fat, high carbs, doesn't matter. Just do NOT drink any calories. All calories must come from food. NOTE: 2 beers or a glass of wine is not the end of the world for a cheat/refeed day. But don't chug regular soda or milkshakes just because it's a cheat day.

5. Once you've hit the calorie limit, it's over. STOP eating and start chugging water. After the cheat meal/refeed, you need to wait as long as you can before eating again.

I know I previously said I don't care if you eat 1 meal a day or 6 meals a day. That's true for every day except the day after a cheat/refeed day.

On the day after a cheat/refeed day, I want you to wait at least 20 hours before eating again.

So let's say you have your cheat/refeed meal on a Sunday. Let's say you end up eating from 6pm to 10pm.

After 10pm , you're done eating and you should not consume any calories until at least 6pm on Monday. If you can wait a full 24 hours, that would be even better.

The idea here is that we've given your body a massive load of calories and carbohydrates during the cheat day, all of which will spike insulin.

Now we want to give the body a chance to process all of that and clear it out of your system before we resume eating. So we're going to take a break from eating for 20-24 hours after the cheat day.

Drink lots of water, as you may find the hunger pangs coming back on the day after the cheat day. Don't give in. One day back on the normal diet and you'll be all fixed up.

After the 20-24 hours have passed, you can have your usual 1,250 calories. Most people prefer to have a lower carbohydrate/higher fat day of eating the day after a cheat day.

If you are weighing yourself on a daily basis, it will probably take 2-3 days to clear out the water weight/salt accumulated during the cheat day.

Days 15-28: The Next Two Weeks

After your first cheat/refeed day, you'll hop back on the diet for another 2 week stretch. Again, nothing brand new here. Still sticking with 1,250 calories per day.

Once you've completed another 13 low-calorie days, you will once again have a cheat/refeed day on the 14th day (28th day overall.)

Same rules as before – keep calories at roughly 2,500 – 3,000 on the cheat/refeed meal and try to eat only one main meal on your cheat/refeed day.

At this point, you'll have completed 4 weeks on The Underground Fat Loss Method. In the next chapter, we'll talk about taking stock of your results after the first 4 week and determining where to go next.

After The First 4 Weeks

After you've finished the first 4 weeks of the diet program, it's time to take stock and formulate a plan moving forward.

At this point there will be 3 possible options:

Option #1: If after the first 4 weeks you are still fatter than you'd like AND you are still above 10% body fat,(for men, 20% for women) then continue with the plan in the usual manner.   1 Cheat/Refeed Meal every 2 weeks. Continue to follow the plan as it was laid out in the previous chapters.

Option #2: If after the first 4 week you are now at 10% body fat (or 20% for women) or less, but you still wish to get leaner still... then continue with the plan at the same calorie level HOWEVER you can now have 1 Cheat/Refeed Meal every week (rather than every 2 weeks.)

This is because leaner people need more frequent refeeds.

Option #3: If after the first 4 weeks you are now at 10% body fat or less (20% for women) and you do NOT desire to get any leaner, then it's time to move to maintenance mode.

The way we handle maintenance is a little different than most so the entire next chapter will be devoted to maintenance.

Note: Men should not try to go any lower than 6% body fat. So the goal of the maintenance program is to keep you at 6-8% body fat without feeling like you're on a diet for the rest of your life.

Women should not go any lower than 12% body fat. The goal of this program for women is to maintain 12-15% bodyfat without feeling like you're on a diet.

Maintenance Mode

Let's be honest: There's no point in getting lean unless you can find a way to maintain it.

After all, getting down to super lean levels only to immediately reverse direction and get fat again is really just a waste of time. And yet, that's what happens to almost everybody. Even professional bodybuilders routinely balloon- up immediately following a contest.

They will often spend 16-20 weeks dieting down to ultra-low body fat levels, then immediately binge for 4 weeks after the contest only to find themselves needing to embark on another 16-20 weeks of dieting in time for the next show.

In this chapter, I'll show you a better way.

You Can't Get Fat In 3 Days

Once you get lean – truly lean (single digit body fat for men, 12-15% for women) then the goods new is you can pig out without gaining a single ounce of body fat.

This was demonstrated in 2014 study out of Fukuoko University. Lean & healthy Japanese men were fed 1,500 calories OVER maintenance for 3 days.

Their body weight and composition was measured before and after the 3 day over- feeding period. After 3 days, the subjects total body weight went up – due to an increase in water weight. But actual amount of body fat stayed the same or even went down in a few cases.

Of course, we know from previous studies that if an overweight person took part in a similar 3-day overfeeding binge, many of the excess calories would be stored as fat.

Why Maintenance Fails

We suck at maintenance. You, me, people in general – we all suck at maintenance. Ever known somebody who lost a bunch of weight with an Atkins (low-carb) approach?

What happened after they went off the diet? Chances are, they gained weight.

And this happens with nearly any diet plan you can think of. The diet works... but then you go off the diet and when you do you gain all the weight back.

The solution is obvious...

Just Don't Go Off The Diet! Stay with me on this. The strategy I'm going to share with you now is controversial.

You've probably never heard anyone talk about this strategy before. And at first it might fly directly in the face of what you THINK a maintenance plan should look like.

But this will be an absolute game-changer for you once you put this strategy into motion so hear me out.

Maintenance level calories for your average adult male will be about 2,250 to 2,500 calories per day. And as I previously explained, by setting our daily calorie target at 1,250 per day, we're creating a massive deficit which will cause rapid weight loss.

Once you achieve you desired leanness, conventional wisdom states that you should then increase your daily caloric target and just start eating 2,250 to 2,500 calories per day. But I'm telling you now if you do that you will just get fat.

Here's what you should do instead:

Rather than abandoning the low-calorie days completely, increase your protein levels slightly so that your new low-calorie daily target is 1,500 calories per day.

You'll do this by taking exactly what you eat for your previous low-calorie days of 1,250 and simply adding 250 calories from lean protein. So you could add an extra serving of tuna fish, or a protein shake or whatever you prefer.

Essentially, this is the same as the "micro-cheat" strategy which will be mentioned in a future chapter.

By this point, you'll have adjusted to the diet and you'll have learned how to successfully manage hunger so the thought of eating only 1,500 calories per day should be simple enough.

But because you are no longer trying to lose weight, you can now employ 2-3 cheat days/meals PER WEEK.

And you can go a little higher on your cheat days/meals. Where before we capped the cheats at 2,500 – 3,000 calories per day, now we can go as high as 3,500 calories per day.

Again, the same rules would apply on the cheat days – try to consolidate the calories to a single window or time-frame (instead of spacing them out throughout the day) and try to always follow up a cheat day/meal with a fast of 20 hours or so to give your body time to manage the influx of calories and carbs.

This means you'd want to avoid having back-to-back cheat days if at all possible.

But I also understand that you if you go to Vegas or NYC for the weekend you'd probably WANT to have back-to-back cheat days.

So go right ahead for special circumstances. As long as you have enough low calorie days before and after the trip, you can get away with quite a lot of "dietary damage" and still stay extremely lean.

So to recap: The key to maintenance is never technically go "off" the diet.

Continue to have low calorie days (recommended at 1,500 calories per day.) Mix in 2-3 higher calorie cheat days of 3,500 calories per day which will allow you to live a "normal" life and still maintain single digit body fat.

A Collection Of Advanced Tips

In this chapter I'll give you a collection of advanced tips and techniques to make your journey towards single-digit body fat faster and easier.

Keep in mind, any of these individual tips are to be considered optional.

Some of these tips are more extreme than others. Don't feel that you must employ any of these tactics, these are all optional and the bulk of your results will come from following the main UFLM plan.

Tip: Veggie, 1 Fruit

Every day (assuming you are not fasting – we'll talk about this later), strive to consume 1 serving of vegetables and 1 serving of fruit.

This will go a long way towards getting you the nutrients you need even on a low-calorie diet like this one.

Tip: Yes, You Can Have A Beer

Yes, alcohol can actually SPEED UP your fat loss.

Here's how:

Often times when I'm shooting for 1,250 calories per day, I find it's easier to just eat one main meal at night.

So I don't eat all day and then I have one massive feast beginning at 8pm each night.

By the time 8pm rolls around... I'm pretty freakin' hungry. So when the clock strikes 8pm.... here's what happens.

Either: I immediately start stuffing my face with pop-tarts, cookies and a bunch of other unhealthy options.

Or

I calmly start cooking a healthy meal based around meat, protein and vegetables. No matter how long it takes to prepare the meal, I am completely relaxed and content.

Option A sounds pretty typical, right? But option B sounds like a proven formula for losing weight.

Luckily, I have a simple trick I use that makes more of my days look like option B.

I use alcohol.

Yup. I've found that when the clock strikes 8pm, if I reward myself with a nice glass of red wine or a nice craft beer... it almost instantly "knocks down" the hunger pangs and allows me to calmly and casually prepare a healthy meal without feeling like I'm starving or suffering.

I don't do this every night, mind you.

Of course, most fitness experts and personal trainers will tell you to avoid alcohol if you want to lose weight. And in theory, they are correct. But in the real world, I've found that alcohol can be a useful tool for achieving your fitness goals.

The keys, of course, are moderation -both with your alcohol consumption and your food consumption.

This plan would not work nearly as well if I was eating all day long and then adding alcohol on top of my food intake. It works because the alcohol allows me to restrict my caloric intake without suffering.

Tip: Nicotine Gum

Ok, obviously this tip is going to be highly controversial but a lot of fitness competitors use this strategy so it's something you should know about. Even if you never put it into action.

Everybody knows smoking is bad for you and highly addictive. But there's a reason why so in Hollywood and modeling industries still smoke – because it kills your appetite.

There's a way to get all the appetite-suppressing qualities of nicotine without lighting up – just chew nicotine gum.

I would avoid using this strategy for more than 2-3 weeks at a time – perhaps reserving this for a short term fat loss "sprint" right before vacation or a special event when you need to maximize fat loss.

Try just 1-2 pieces per day and start with the lowest available dosage (usually 1 mg.) You should get a slight buzz (similar to caffeine buzz) and it should curb your appetite. If you don't feel anything, you may need to try a higher dosage. And if you feel nauseas, at a higher dosage then you may need to drop down to a lower level.

Tip: Weigh Yourself Every Day

I learned this one from a reclusive tech millionaire who sold his company and moved to the Swiss alps. The man was a genius, but could never seem to figure out how to crack the weight loss code.

Then he decided to view weight loss the same way a computer engineer would view any computer problem – he "hacked it."

Essentially he figured out what I've already told you – that to lose weight you need to drastically cut your calories. But he also employed an interesting feedback loop. He weighed himself every day and plotted the data.

The act of weighing yourself every day forces you to stay honest with yourself. And even though you won't see the numbers on the scale get smaller every day, over time you'll see a downward trend.

Tip: Red Licorice For Fat Loss

Obviously, candy is not a great choice if you're trying to get lean and control your caloric intake.

But I understand you probably can't swear off candy forever. So if you're faced with a situation where you need to eat some candy, opt for licorice.

It's virtually fat free --- since fat has the most calories per gram of any other macronutrient you can control calories simply by avoiding foods that are high in fat. Most candy is high in fat AND carbs (which is why candy is delicious.) And while licorice is high in carbs, it's virtually fat free.

Plus black licorice – if you can stomach it – actually contains a compound called glycyrrhetinic acid that's been shown in studies to increase fat burning. Obviously licorice is certainly not a magic pill, but if find yourself reaching for candy, you may as well reach for licorice.

Tip: Dirty Dreams For Faster Fat Loss

Get more sleep – it's advice that we all ignore. But for those trying to lose fat, it's crucial. For two reasons:

First, lack of sleep reduces your willpower. Making it more likely to fall off the wagon. But second, the more you sleep the less you need to rely on willpower.

Think about it: If you stay up until midnight, that means you've probably got 2-3 hours where you're most likely watching TV or messing around on the internet and likely to be tempted by whatever is in the cupboard.

But if you go to sleep at 10pm, you don't have to fight that battle. Of course, sometimes it can be tougher to fall asleep when you're dieting. To that end, here are a couple supplements that seem to help with sleep issues.

The first is melatonin – probably not a big surprise for anyone reading this. Start with the lowest dose you can find, and then take one pill/tablet about 30 minutes before bed.

Another recommendation is Valerian Root. I've found this supplement not only relaxes you before bed time.

As an added bonus, a lot of people say that valerian root actually gives them "dirty" dreams (yup, talkin' 'about sex stuff here) so it you needed another reason to hit the sheets early, that should do it.

Tip: Make Your Exercise In-Efficient

There's a cruel lesson that most people who train for marathons end up learning along the way. Training and running 26.2 miles is not a great way to get lean.

For starters, running 26.2 miles only burns about 2,800 calories. Which means you can actually "undo" that workout with a single cheat day.

Are you shocked at how few calories get burned up from such a herculean task? Most people are.

Because we tend to believe things that are hard burn a lot of calories. But the truth is the human body has adapted to conserve calories. So the more you run, the more your body finds ways to efficiently preserve calories.

That's why it's nearly impossible to create a big caloric deficit via exercise and that's why we use diet to create a big deficit instead.

Tip: Smash Through The Cycle Of Sadness

There's something that happens when you start a diet. The first two weeks go great, and you can actually see positive results on almost a daily basis.

Yes, you're burning fat but you're also dropping a lot of water weight in that first week or two. After the first two weeks, the results start to lose down a bit. And to make matters worse, you can can't control where your body burns fat.

So while it's fun when your body is burning fat from your stomach areas, you can start to lose your mind a little bit when the fat comes off your arms (making your arms look smaller).

I've heard it referred to as "The Dark Period" and I think that sums it up. Starting a diet is usually rewarding because you see quick results. And being lean is awesome.   But it's the space in-between is what causes most people to fail.

When you are in the "dark period" you might be tempted to change courses, completely abandon your strategy and throw in the towel and blame you genetics.

If you do that, you'll be stuck forever. You'll start a diet, quit, start another diet, quit... and on and on forever.

The solution is to smash through the dark period. Refuse to quit just because you 'feel' like the diet isn't working. (This is why the previous tip about weighing yourself daily and keeping an accurate log is important.)

In business we say one data point is better than a thousand opinions. When you feel like a diet isn't working, that's an opinion.

When you look in the mirror and you think you're losing muscle... that's an opinion.

That's why it's important to measure your results and stay the course even when you're making your way through the dark period.

Tip: Micro-cheats

This is an advanced strategy that most guys probably won't even need. First, this is for guys who are in single-digit body fat territory but trying to get leaner.

On some days your body will just demand more food. You'll know it when it happens because by the time you get to single-digit body fat, you've trained yourself to differentiate between actual hunger and "mental" hunger.

So on these rare days (again, this is only for guys already in single digit body fat and even then you'll only need to do this 1 or 2 times per month MAX) just consume an additional 250 calories from LEAN protein only. Essentially, some extra chicken or tuna fish.

This will immediately blunt your hunger and as an added bonus you'll often see a rapid response as your muscles will seem to "soak up" the added protein and you'll look bigger and stronger almost right away.

Foods For Fat Loss

There are no truly "magic" foods for fat loss. However, there are some foods that provide a very high level of nutrients with a low level of calories and for our purposes, that's pretty close to magical.

In this chapter I'll give you a collection of foods that can help you achieve your single-digit body fat goals. Most of the people I know who've achieved single digit body fat end up eating foods from this list quite often.

Greek Yogurt: This stuff is a godsend as far as I'm concerned. I get the big tub from Kroger.

A full tub of the Kroger Vanilla Greek Yogurt has 3 cups and provides just 420 calories, but with 63 grams of protein, only 39 grams of carbs and just 1.5 grams of fat. This is one my preferred foods on a low- fat/higher carb day.

If you don't live near a Kroger, I've also found the plain Greek yogurt from Costco provides a comparable alternative.

Tuna Fish: 2 (4oz) cans of tuna fish (packed in water) give you 44 grams of protein with just 200 calories and only 2 grams of fat. (0 carbs.) I don't love the taste of tuna fish, but the nutrient profile is so good I often eat this on my lower carb days.

I'll put some lettuce on a plate, open and drain 2 cans of tuna, put the tuna on the lettuce, top with bacon bits and some lite Italian dressing and you've got a decent meal that gives you plenty of protein with very few calories. This is very filling.

Potato: The potato is a very under-rated diet food as far as I'm concerned. White potatoes have gotten a bad rap over the years because they've been lumped into the same category as white bread.

But potatoes are incredibly filling and low in calories which is perfect for our purposes. A large Russett potato contains roughly 110 calories and you'd be surprised how full you can get from a single potato.

Here's what I do: I take a large potato and poke a few holes in it with a fork. Put the potato on a microwaveable plate.

On the same plate I put a mug of water. Then put potato and mug in the microwave on high for 5 minutes.
This is essentially the "lazy" way to bake a potato in just about 5 minutes.

Once it gets out of the microwave I'll chop it up and add it to some scrambled eggs with salsa.

Egg Whites: I used to be a big fan of whole eggs but I've found that when trying to lose weight you need to cut calories wherever you can.

So for that reason, I've grown fond of egg whites. 2 cups of liquid egg whites give you just 240 calories, along with 20 grams of protein and only 4 carbs.

I'll usually take my eggs scrambled using 1 TBSP of butter in a pan, 2 cups of egg whites and 1 slice of American cheese. In total this provides a very filling 412 calories.

Add the aforementioned potato and salsa and you've got a very decent meal for only 600 calories.

Red Wine: Often times the key to successfully staying with a diet is to avoid the feeling that you are "on a diet." For this reason, I've found a glass of red wine to be a very valuable dieting tool.

For a few reasons: First, if you're in a social situation you can have a glass of red wine and appear "normal" to the outside world.

Even if you are at a dinner party, if you abstain from all food and only have water, it appears strange.

But if you abstain from all food and say that you're just not hungry WHILE still having a glass of red wine, suddenly that's much more normal in the eyes of others.

In addition, I've found that a glass of red wine can be a valuable tool to blunt your appetite.

Often times when I just get home after a long day I find myself ravenously hungry. I could just eat a bunch of food without even thinking about it.

Or I can pour myself a glass of red wine and have a casual and relaxed few minutes. Slowly sipping the red wine seems to completely kill the appetite which allows you to make smarter and better food choices.

And since a glass of red wine contains only 130 calories, the indulgence still leaves you plenty of available calories for food.

Oatmeal: I mentioned previously that I eat oatmeal almost every night to help me sleep. ½ cup of oatmeal, missed with 1 cup of water in a bowl, microwaved for 90 seconds, topped with cinnamon and with 1TBSP of peanut butter swirled in, then I pour a splash of Almond milk on top. Total calories: Just 290 for a very filling late night snack.

Pickles: Practically zero calories and high in salt (which can help you feel full.) I once interviewed a group of people, all of which had lost over 100 pounds.

More than half of them snacked on pickles to lose all the weight.

Hunger

If there is one big "secret" to successfully getting down (and staying) in single-digit body fat, it's learning to deal with hunger.

The average person has an "immature" relationship with hunger. By that I mean the average person views hunger in the exact same way a baby views the need to poop or piss.

When a baby feels the need to empty it's bladder or empty it's bowels, it simply does so immediately.

An adult human with an immature relationship with hunger often reacts in much the same way.

If an adult (overweight) human is driving a car and feels even the slightest twinge of hunger, he or she will immediately pull the car into the nearest fast foods restaurant.

As a baby grows into a toddler, we no longer tolerate their "immature" relationship with the need to poop & pee.

We train our toddlers to DELAY the need to poop & pee until they can get to the toilet.

An adult may feel the need to urinate, but can often delay for hours if needs be. Because he's been trained to do so.

Yet this very same adult – who now has a "mature" relationship with his bowel function – can still have an immature relationship with hunger.

To achieve single-digit body fat, you simply need to train your response to hunger.

When you get hungry, it is normal to recognize and be aware of the sensation of hunger.

Acknowledge it. And understand that you can eat... just not right now.

Hunger will scream at you: "Eat now or you'll die!"

You need to be smarter than that. Hunger is a vicious sensation.

Humans have literally been driven mad from hunger, even cut off their own fingers when in the grasps of true starvation.

But you need to recognize the difference between feeling "a little bit peckish" and true starvation.

True starvation occurs after multiple WEEKS without food. Not after a few hours.

You are in command of your body. You are the captain.

My friend in the fitness industry "J-Max" once told me a story about delivering groceries to a woman who was nearly 100 years old... but didn't look a day over 65.

She told him her "secret" was to embrace hunger.

She told him many years ago she realized that "hunger is what it feels like to be lean."

To the average overweight person, that sounds like lunacy. But the average overweight person is absolutely terrified of the sensation of hunger.

The person who successfully gets and stays lean recognizes that to do so you must embrace hunger.

Hunger is not something to be feared. Hunger is a valuable tool. Hunger increases productivity.

When you are hungry, your body is actively breaking down stored calories (fat) to provide the energy you need to continue your day.

Our ancestors many years ago had developed a mature relationship with hunger.

Not every hunt was successful. Not every harvest yielded a full bounty of crops. So hunger wasn't such a foreign concept to humans in years past.

I will leave you with this last thought regarding hunger the art of delaying gratification. On this plan you can have any food you want... in any amounts you want. Just not always WHEN you want.   If you think about it, that's a pretty good deal.

Over the course of a full week, you could be eating many of the same foods that a 300 pound massively obese person eats, perhaps in the same quantities as well.

While you'll enjoy walking around with single-digit body fat while the overweight person may never figure out how to lose weight.

So one more time: Embrace hunger. Hunger is the key that unlocks the door to leanness.

Loss Of Muscle, Loss Of Testosterone & The Monster Under The Bed

When it comes to getting lean, there are a few "monsters under the bed" that tend to trip up most men.

I call them "monsters under the bed" because they are not real. They are imaginary. And yet, just as an imaginary monster under the bed can cause a very real loss of sleep for a child, these imaginary threats can derail many guys who otherwise would end up with single-digit body fat.

So let's slay these imaginary monsters once and for all:

Loss of Muscle: The fitness industry as a whole has created this fear of losing muscle and blown it way out of proportion.

Here's the truth: To lose muscle, you must stop using it.

Think about what happens if you break a bone in your arm. The doctor puts your arm in a cast and 8 weeks later when the cast comes off your arm is shriveled and weak.

It doesn't matter if you were over-eating or under-eating – because you were not using the muscles in your arm.

So eating fewer calories does not mean your body will "eat" your muscle.

Another myth that the fitness industry continues to reinforce is the idea that for some reason your body will choose to burn muscle and "hold on" to body fat.

Again, this has no basis in science. Often referred to as the "starvation mode" myth, this has been disproven in military studies.

Military researchers took recruits and essentially ran them into the ground to see what it actually took to get a person into true "starvation mode."

So they had these military guys eating 1,000 calories a day and burning upwards of 6,000 calories a day from exercise!

They discovered guys did not lose muscle UNTIL they reached 5-6% body fat. (This is why I don't recommend guys try to get any leaner than 6% body fat.)

To understand why the body works like this, you need to understand a little bit about how stored body fat works.

If you have 50 pounds of excess body fat on your body and you start to cut your calories, your body will turn to the stored calories (body fat) to provide energy.

This makes sense when you think about it. The primary purpose of this stored body fat is to provide calories when food is scarce.

If the body "decided" to burn muscle mass instead of body fat, it wouldn't make any sense from an evolutionary perspective.

If muscle was sacrificed, it would make you slower and weaker which would negatively impact your hunting skills and make it even MORE difficult to acquire food.

But by burning body fat and sparing muscle, it makes you leaner, lighter and faster – thus INCREASING your chances of having a successful hunt.

This holds true for losing body fat UNTIL you get to about 5% body fat. At this point, you will only have a few pounds of body fat left and this remaining body fat will be the fat surrounding your organs.

This fat is very valuable because it shields and protects your organs – it is essential for maintaining life.

Even though the body does not "want" to burn muscle, when there is no longer any "extra" body fat to burn and the only remaining body fat is the fat surrounding your organs, the body will then at that point burn muscle in an attempt to save the organs and preserve life.

So long story short, if you are at 6% body fat and trying to get leaner, loss of muscle might be a concern.

If you are at 19% body fat and concerned that skipping breakfast might cause you to suddenly lose all your muscle, you're being ridiculous.

Loss of Testosterone

The next big fear that guys have is that dieting or simply the process of losing body fat will cause a reduction in testosterone levels.

This is interesting because there is actually a little bit of truth to this statement... but perhaps not how you think.

Studies show that men with more body fat have higher levels of estrogen (since body fat breeds estrogen) and lower levels of testosterone. So you might think that losing body fat would cause a rise in testosterone levels.

And that does indeed happen – eventually.

But the PROCESS of losing body fat can actually cause a TEMPORARY reduction in testosterone levels. Again, this is only TEMPORARY. Here's proof:

A 1987 study had men doing a 10-day water-only fast.

The first day after the fast they were allowed to eat 1,500 calories and then after that they ate normally for 4 days.

As you might expect, eating zero food or calories for 10 days did in fact cause testosterone levels to drop.

No a big surprise there.

But as you can see from the chart, the testosterone levels dropped only slightly and actually soared ABOVE their original levels once the men resumed eating.

On the Underground Fat Loss program, we will NOT be fasting for 10 days or anything like that. So we would expect any dip in testosterone would be minor by comparison.

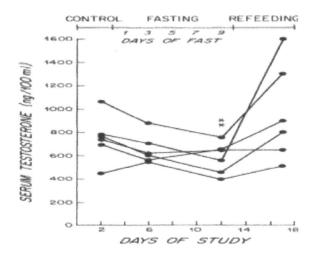

And if you actually finish the plan and get down to your goal level of leanness and then get to the point where you are enjoying 2-3 refeed days per week, it's quite possible you could end up with the highest testosterone levels of your life thanks to your new lean physique.

So stop worrying about losing muscle or lower testosterone levels – as I've just shown you those fears are largely unfounded.

Start the plan and see it through until you hit your goal.

Family, Friends & Other Obstacles

Let me tell you a story. About a guy named Bobby.
Bobby has an idea for a business. He is standing in front of
two rooms.

On his left is a room full of Bobby's friends, neighbors and
co-workers. On this right, a room full of wildly successful
self-made business people.

If Bobby walks into the room with his friends and neighbors
and tells them about his plan to go into business for
himself... do you know what will happen?

They will laugh at him. Cut him down. Try to reason with
him. Or give him condescending offerings of hope.

If Bobby walks into the room with self-made business
people and tells them about his plans, do you know what
will happen? They'll will encourage, advise and perhaps
even mentor him.

Which is somewhat strange if you think about it. If Bobby
becomes a big success, his success could threaten their
existing businesses. Yet on the other hand, if Bobby's
business becomes a success, his friends and family are likely
to reap many of the rewards.

So why would the already established business people be willing to encourage him... while his friends and family try to drag him down?

It makes absolutely no sense... and yet the exact same things happens when trying to get in shape.

Find somebody who's already in great shape and tell them you're trying to lose a few pounds or get in better shape. They'll probably offer to help.

And yet, if you share your plans with a family member, a friend or a co-worker I can predict with almost uncanny certainty what will happen next. Best case: They'll mock you.

That is literally the best case scenario. Because it's far more likely that your friends and family members will actively sabotage you.

Even if they support you from the jump, once you start making progress there's a good chance you'll start hearing comments about how you're "too skinny" now or they'll be begging you to eat more.

What they're really saying is "stop improving yourself because every incremental improvement makes me feel exponentially worse about myself. And change is difficult so I'd rather you stop improving."

Make no mistake about it: When you improve yourself – in any way – in may appear to be a harmless activity. But in reality, you end up becoming a MIRROR to those around you.

They don't look at you and see... well, you. They look at you and see a reflection of themselves. They look at you and see what could be done if they could will themselves to make a change.

But alas, most people cannot change. Most people cannot delay gratification for even a moment and so they feel trapped inside their own skin. Most days, they're fine with it.

As long as they remain surrounded by other powerless people. But once you break free, once you rise above and demonstrate your ability to change and grow... then they'll turn their hatred towards you.

So what is the solution? Must you abandon your co-workers, your friends and your family? Of course not. But you must steel yourself against their comments and their actions.

Nobody is going to hold you down and pour gravy down your throat. They don't force you to get or remain fat. But they'll beg, whine, cajole. So you must change your stance.

You have to change who you are from the core.

The captain of an army does not pay any mind to the grumbles of the foot soldiers. You too must see yourself as the leader, as the captain. Blaze your own path.

If others around you choose to support you, welcome them with open arms. But if they do not, it makes no difference as you're quite happy to travel this journey alone.

Parting Words

That's it. There is nothing else to read. Put this plan into action and drop me a line once you reach your goals.

Will it be easy? No. It will not. But once you've achieved your goal I believe you'll look back and realize it was far easier than you thought it would be.

I've already given you everything you need to get started with this plan. But to make your journey even easier, I'm including the following resources:

1: What I Ate
2: Recommended Workouts
3: Recommended Supplements.
4: How To Burn 3x More Fat In The Next 48 Hours

What I Ate

In this chapter, I'm going to show you screen grabs from my MyFitnessPal app.

I'll include my comments AFTER each screen grab. Please use this as examples of what 1 person ate on this diet. Do NOT feel that you have to copy these meals exactly.

Breakfast	Calories	Carbs	Fat	Protein	Sodium	Sugar	
Add Food | Quick Tools							
Lunch							
Add Food | Quick Tools							
Dinner							
Cucumber - With peel, raw, 1 cucumber (8-1/4")	45	11	0	2	6	5	
Kroger - American Cheese Single Slices, 1 slice (19g)	70	0	5	4	200	0	
Egg - Beaters, 1.5 cup	180	3	0	15	225	0	
Butter - Unsalted, 1 tbsp	102	0	12	0	2	0	
Home Made - Taco Meat - All Natural Ground Beef 80/20 and Casa Mamita Seasoning, 4 oz	313	19	22	19	630	0	
Jiffy - Creamy Peanut Butter, 1 Tablespoon	95	4	8	4	0	2	
Silk - Pure Almond Milk (Vanilla), 8 oz	90	16	3	1	160	15	
Kroger - Oatmeal, 1/2 cup cooked	150	27	3	6	0	1	
Woolworths - Mini Cup Cake, 1 cake	84	25	4	2	68	14	
Russel - Potatoe, 1 potato	110	26	0	3	0	1	
Add Food | Quick Tools	1,239	131	56	55	1,291	38	

Comments: This is pretty typical lower-carb day for me. I want you to notice that even though I was not "perfect" (I happily scarfed down a mini-cupcake with my daughter while drinking pretend tea at an impromptu tea party) I still came in under my calorie target of 1,250 calories per day.

The food selection might look a little confusing on paper, but essentially what I do is when I get home from work, I eat my veggies first (cucumber).

While I'm eating that, I'm making scrambled eggs with the egg beaters, cheese & butter. While I'm cooking that I "bake" a potato in the microwave for 5 minutes, and warm up the taco meat (previously cooked.)

Then I put the scrambled eggs, taco meat and diced potato in a bowl and cover with salsa. All in all, a very satisfying meal.

Before bed I'll have the oatmeal with peanut butter and almond milk as a pre-bed snack. (Helps me sleep).

Breakfast	Calories	Carbs	Fat	Protein	Sodium	Sugar	
Add Food | Quick Tools							
Lunch							
Add Food | Quick Tools							
Dinner							
Cucumber - With peel, raw, 1 cucumber (8-1/4")	45	11	0	2	6	5	●
Meijer - Chunk Light Tuna Fish In Water, 2 container (4 oz (drained) ea.)	200	0	2	44	720	0	●
Lettuce - Romaine Lettuce, 2 cups	20	4	0	2	20	4	●
bacos - Bacon Bits, 1.5 tbs	30	2	1	3	115	1	●
Kroger - Oatmeal, 1/2 cup cooked	150	27	3	6	0	1	●
Silk - Pure Almond Milk (Vanilla), 8 oz	90	16	3	1	160	15	●
Jify - Creamy Peanut Butter, 1 Tablespoon	95	4	8	4	0	2	●
Kraft - Life house italian, 6 tbso	105	15	3	0	930	6	●
Sims - Beef Snack Sticks, 6 stick (16g)	360	0	30	18	1,200	0	●
Add Food | Quick Tools	1,095	79	49	79	3,151	34	

Comments: Another lower-carb day. Notice I would certainly not call these "low" carb days, just "lower" as in "lower" than how most people eat.

This is good meal template for when you don't feel like cooking. I just put the tuna fish (from cans) on a bed of lettuce, add some bacon bits and some Italian dressing.

I eat the beef sticks afterwards as a snack. And then again I have the oatmeal as a pre-bed snack.

Breakfast	Calories	Carbs	Fat	Protein	Sodium	Sugar	
Add Food | Quick Tools							
Lunch							
Add Food | Quick Tools							
Dinner							
Generic - Banana **, 1 Banana (126g)	110	30	0	1	0	19	⊖
Kelloggs - Chocolate Fudge Pop Tart, 1 Pastry	200	37	5	3	230	19	⊖
Kroger - Greek All Natural Nonfat Vanilla Yogurt, 3 cup (227g)	420	39	2	63	315	36	⊖
Kroger Vanilla Flavored Flakes With Almonds - Cereal, 1 1/2 cup	220	50	3	4	300	18	⊖
Silk - Pure Almond Milk (Vanilla), 8 oz	90	16	3	1	160	15	⊖
Kroger - Oatmeal, 1/2 cup cooked	150	27	3	6	0	1	⊖
Jiffy - Creamy Peanut Butter, 1 Tablespoon	95	4	8	4	0	2	⊖
Add Food | Quick Tools	1,285	203	23	82	1,005	110	

Comments: As I mentioned before, I like to do 2 "lower carb" days followed by a "higher carb" day. This is primarily for mental sanity (nobody wants to eat the same foods day in a day out).

As you can see, this is another good template for those that hate cooking. And as you can see, I wasn't perfect.

I should not have had that pop-tart, but I still came in very close to my target of 1,250 calories per day.

Breakfast	Calories	Carbs	Fat	Protein	Sodium	Sugar
Add Food | Quick Tools						
Lunch						
Add Food | Quick Tools						
Dinner						
Kroger - Oatmeal, 1/2 cup cooked	150	27	3	6	0	1
Jify - Creamy Peanut Butter, 1 Tablespoon	95	4	8	4	0	2
Hungry Howies - Large Sausage Pizza, 4 slice	904	103	27	54	464	0
Add Food | Quick Tools	1,149	134	38	64	464	3

Comments: Sometimes, you will want or need to eat like a normal person just because you can't always eat tuna or egg whites.

This day shows a good example of how to handle that. This is also why I prefer to eat just one large meal per day (in the evening) most days because I can get away with eating 4 pizzas of pizza and still end up well below my calorie target.

On this day we ended up going out for pizza. Rather than sit at the table eating nothing (and looking like an oddball) I just ate a few slices of pizza. Nobody would think that I was "on a diet" but by limiting the damage I was able to still come in under my target for the day.

Breakfast

Add Food | Quick Tools

Lunch

Add Food | Quick Tools

Dinner

	Calories	Carbs	Fat	Protein	Sodium	Sugar	
Generic - Banana **, 1 Banana (126g)	110	30	0	1	0	19	⊖
Kelloggs - Chocolate Fudge Pop Tart, 1 Pastry	200	37	5	3	230	19	⊖
Kroger - Greek All Natural Nonfat Vanilla Yogurt, 3 cup (227g)	420	39	2	63	315	36	⊖
Kroger Vanilla Flavored Flakes With Almonds - Cereal, 1 1/2 cup	220	50	3	4	300	18	⊖
Silk - Pure Almond Milk (Vanilla), 8 oz	90	16	3	1	160	15	⊖
Kroger - Oatmeal, 1/2 cup cooked	150	27	3	6	0	1	⊖
Jiffy - Creamy Peanut Butter, 1 Tablespoon	95	4	8	4	0	2	⊖
Add Food	Quick Tools	1,285	203	23	82	1,005	110	

Comments: Here's an example of a higher-carb/lower fat day. On days where I feel the need for more protein, I'll usually just skip the cereal and instead opt for a double-serving of Greek yogurt which gets me 120 grams of protein.

Breakfast	Calories	Carbs	Fat	Protein	Sodium	Sugar	
Eas Rtd - Advantage - Chocolate Fudge, 11 fl oz	110	5	3	17	470	0	⊖
Add Food | Quick Tools	110	5	3	17	470	0	

Lunch							
Jets - Deep Dish Pepperoni Pizza, 1 slice	324	30	15	16	518	1	⊖
Add Food | Quick Tools	324	30	15	16	518	1	

Dinner							
Kroger - Oatmeal, 1/2 cup cooked	150	27	3	6	0	1	⊖
Jify - Creamy Peanut Butter, 1 Tablespoon	95	4	8	4	0	2	⊖
Kroger - American Cheese Single Slices, 1 slice (19g)	70	0	5	4	200	0	⊖
Butter - Unsalted, 1 tbsp	102	0	12	0	2	0	⊖
Egg - Beaters, 2 cup	240	4	0	20	300	0	⊖
Silk - Pure Almond Milk (Vanilla), 8 oz	90	16	3	1	160	15	⊖
Kroger - White Chicken Chili, 0.5 cup	115	0	0	0	0	0	⊖
Cucumber - With peel, raw, 1 cucumber (8-1/4")	45	11	0	2	6	5	⊖
Russel - Potatoe, 1 potato	110	26	0	3	0	1	⊖
Add Food | Quick Tools	1,017	88	38	40	668	24	

Comments: Lastly, I want to show that you do NOT need to eat only 1 meal per day, as is my preferred method. In this example, I actually had a protein shake for breakfast, pizza for lunch and dinner at home and STILL stayed WAY under my calorie target of 1,250 per day.

So 1 meal a day or 3, it doesn't really matter. Do what works best for you.

Recommended Workouts

People constantly ask me about the best "workout" to burn fat. But that's really the wrong question. That's like asking what's the best car to drive if you want to get from New York to Paris.

Losing weight and burning fat is all about the DIET, which I've just shown. Resistance training IS important, but simply because resistance training helps burn and maintain muscle – you actually burn very calories during a resistance training workout.

Cardio-based training is wholly in-efficient because a) it takes time, b) you never burn as many calories as you think and
c) often times cardio training just makes you hungrier.

So when it comes to the "best" type of workout for burning fat, there are 3 truths you need to recognize.

The first truth is you need to focus on resistance-training workouts.

The second truth is that the specific TYPE of resistance-training workout you follow doesn't really matter. It's the diet that drives your results, not the workouts.

The third and perhaps most surprising truth – you need far less "working out" then you think if it's your goal to get lean.

In fact, during a recent time period following this plan I suffered a minor injury that forced me to stop working out for two weeks.

During the previous two weeks, I had a busy period at work and I ended up missing a couple of my regularly scheduled workouts. So over the course of a MONTH I ended up working out just 4 TIMES.

And yet during the entire time I stuck to the diet as planned. The result? I got leaner throughout the month and didn't see any noticeable loss of muscle.

So don't get too caught up trying to find the perfect workout. Find something you like, something you can stick with on a regular basis and try your best to be consistent. But above all else, it's the diet that will get you lean.
Recommended Workout:

DUP stands for "Daily Undulating Periodization" and this workout is geared towards advanced trainers willing to train more often (4-6 times per week) in exchange for better gains in muscle and strength.

It's not for everyone, but if you can get to the gym at least 4x per week and if you're comfortable training squats, bench presses and deadlifts this program will probably give you your fastest gains in muscle and strength.

You can read more about how DUP works with a simple research on internet.

Supplements

If you want you can skip this section all together. You do NOT need any supplements at all for this plan.

However, I get so many questions from people asking what things they can take that will actually help, so here's a short list. You can easily find this supplements on internet:

Multi-vitamin: Already covered in a previous chapter. We're drastically cutting calories on this plan so it makes sense to take a multi-vitamin and make sure your nutrient needs are covered.

I don't think any brand is really superior to the others, but this one is fun because it makes your urine turn all different kinds of colors and some people swear this is the best one so it might be worth trying out.

Creatine: Can help preserve muscle during times of strict dieting. Just get the cheap stuff – creatine monohydrate – and don't expect any miracles.

Protein Powder: I prefer to eat solid food whenever possible as this will always be more filling, but a good low-carb protein powder is always handy in a pinch. This is the brand I use.

Fish Oil: I don't think fish oil is anywhere NEAR as important as people make it out to be.

But some people say it helps with joint pain or existing medical conditions so if you feel better taking fish oil, then continue to do so.

But keep in mind calories from fish oil still count so a tablespoon of most fish oil probably contains 120 calories so be sure to account for that.

Vitamin D: Again, people are making some pretty wild claims about this stuff – most of which I think are ridiculous.

But if like me you A) work in an office, B) have pale skin and C) live in a cold-weather climate where you go without sun for much of the year, it's probably worth taking Vitamin D just to make sure you're not deficient.

Best Fat Loss Supplement: Black coffee.

There are actually quite a few studies showing how caffeine benefits fat loss.
So if you're having trouble dealing with hunger pangs, try a cup of black coffee. Yes, it tastes awful but it does a great job of killing hunger.

And it's cheap!

How To Burn 3x More Fat In The Next 48 Hours

I call this next section "gun to the head" fat loss. This is 100% optional. A friend of mine lost 60 pounds and got down to single-digit body fat just by eating 1,250 calories a day and having a bi-weekly high calorie day. Seriously. That basics work.

However, if you are working with an accelerated time line or if you simply want to lose body fat as fast as possible, then this chapter is for you.

I call it "gun to the head fat loss" because if you put a gun to my head and forced me to lose fat as quickly as possible, I could absolutely incorporate the strategy you'll find in this chapter.

I call this part "The 44 Hour Diet."

The diet plan I'm about to reveal to you sounds like science-fiction. It sounds too good to be true. And yet, the plan is based on science. Most who hear about the plan scoff. But those who actually try it quickly become raving fans.

In just a moment, you'll see why.

And let me tell you.... NOTHING works better for both immediate results and LASTING weight loss than the 44-hour diet. I'm excited for you to experience this for yourself.

But first, let me reveal the science behind why this method works so well...

The Science Behind The 44 Hour Diet
Here are just a few of the scientific reasons why the 44-hour diet plan is so effective:

Forces Your Body To Burn Stored Body Fat 3x Faster... WITHOUT exercise.

Studies show the method behind the 44-hour diet actually burns stored body fat at a rate up to 3x FASTER than traditional diet plans.

Increases growth hormone levels by 500%... naturally.

Have you heard of growth hormone? It's a naturally occurring hormone. When you're young, your body produces high levels of growth hormone. Growth hormone improves your sleep, burns fat, increases lean muscle tissue, controls energy and mood levels and makes your feel younger.

This hormone is so incredible that many wealthy individuals over the age of 45 actually consider this to be a fountain of youth.

In Hollywood, many leading actors and actresses actually shell out upwards of $2,000 a month for synthetic growth hormone injections because it keeps you looking young and vibrant and turns back the clock.

The best and famous actors and actresses praise the drug for restoring their youthfulness and energy levels.

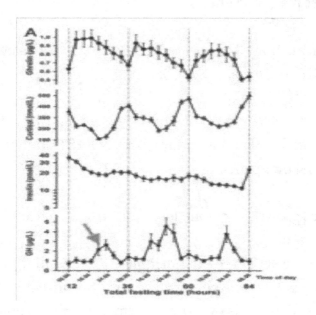

But here's the thing: You don't need to shell out thousands of dollars a month for synthetic growth hormone injections. Because your body produces growth hormone NATURALLY.

And studies show that during the 44-hour diet, your body actually produces 500% more growth hormone.

In addition to that, cortisol (the stress hormone) levels drop. So you will actually feel more at peace and more relaxed even as you're losing weight.

Kills hunger levels

During the 44-hour diet, insulin levels (the hormone that tells your body to store fat) drop. And Ghrelin (the hunger hormone) falls off as well. So even though you only need to stick with the 44-hour diet for a very short period of time, many people find it incredibly easy to follow because they just don't feel hungry.

In fact, unlike traditional diets that make you more hungry the longer you stay on the diet, the 44-hour diet actually gets EASIER near the end because your ghrelin levels continue to fall the entire time.

Regenerate Your Immune System

A study out of the University of Southern California shows that those who followed the principles of the 44-hour diet actually saw remarkable regeneration of their immune systems, including an increase in active white blood cells and a large decrease in the enzyme PKA – which is an enzyme linked to cancer and aging.

Boosts Your Metabolism

Traditionally, your metabolism (or your "resting metabolic rate") actually gets lower when dieting. This is why people regain the weight so quickly after you end the diet.

However, studies show that using the 44-hour diet can actually INCREASE your metabolism/metabolic rate by 14%!

So not only will be burning fat during the 44-hour diet, you'll also boosting your metabolism so you can continue to burn fat during the rest of the week.

More Energy/More Focus/More Freetime

I get more done during my 44-hour diet than I do the rest of the week.

And that's because during the 44-hour diet, I have way more energy, extreme levels of focus and as a result way more free time as compared to the rest of the week.

Are you starting to see why the 44-hour diet can be so incredibly effective?

By this point, you're probably eager to learn exactly what the 44-hour diet is, so in a minute I'll give you the full story. But first...

The True Story Of The Scottish Man Who Lost 293 Pounds
In One Year

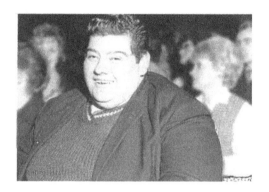

Frank Detomaso once tipped the scales at over 450 pounds.
Like many people, he'd struggled with his weight for his
entire life.

His father owned a popular fish & chip restaurant in his
hometown of Dundee, Scotland.

Frank worked there as a child and continued working there
as an adult.

Surrounded by food all day long at work, and at home as
well, Angus's weight quickly spiraled out of control.

He'd tried diets and exercise before, but nothing seemed to
work. For one reason or another he'd just end up quitting,

gaining even more weight and then trying another diet... quitting, and on and on.

It's a vicious cycle – and even those who only have 10-20 pounds of fat to lose can relate. So in 1965, Frank made the decision that would forever change his life.

He woke up, put on his clothes and walked into the Maryfield hospital in Dundee, Scotland. Frank told the admitting physician that he couldn't live like this anymore and he was prepared to take drastic measure to get his weight under control once and for all.

Soon, a team of doctors gathered around Frank. He had but one question: "What would happen if a man simply stopped eating?"

"For how long?" The doctors asked. Frank replied. "For as long as it takes."

Realizing what Frank was proposing, the doctors strongly advised against it. Frank was asking about a long-term fast for the purposes of losing fat. "You could die" the doctors warned.

But Frank had already made his mind up before he'd walked into the hospital that day. And the doctors could do nothing to change his resolve.

Realizing that Frank was hell-bent on his plan, the doctors urged him to at least check in with them on a regular basis so they could monitor his health.

Frank agreed and he became the star subject of a long-term study on fasting. For the next 392 days, Frank lived his life as normal. He worked, he read, he laughed... he did all the things a normal person would do.

Except... that he didn't eat. No solid food and his only drinks were water, coffee and tea. 392 days later, Frank broke his fast with a hardboiled egg and piece of toast. For the first time in perhaps his entire life... such a small amount of food gave Frank a feeling he'd never had before.

He felt full.

A few years later, the Guinness Book of World Records recognized Frank Detomas's feat and awarded his the record for the longest fast. Frank ended up losing almost 300 pounds during his ordeal – nearly a pound per day.

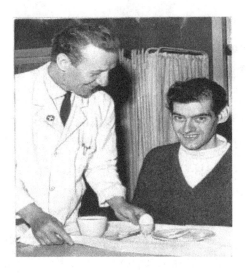

What amazes researchers is that he suffered virtually zero ill effects from such an extreme undertaking.

Perhaps even more amazing, Frank never attempted another such fast and yet he successfully kept the weight off for the rest of his life. He married, raised two children and died decades later after a long and fulfilling life.

9,408 Hours Without Food

In total, Frank Detomaso went 9,408 hours without food. I'm breaking it out by the hour because the diet plan I'm about to reveal to you will seem like a drop in the bucket by comparison.

You can burn fat, eat all of your favorite foods, get lean and stay lean... if you're willing to fast for the first 44 hours of the week – that's less than a half a single percent of the time that Frank Detomaso did.

While I realize you may have never gone more than a few hours without food before and that what I'm proposing might sound drastically different than anything you've done before, don't worry.

You CAN do this.

I have hundreds of emails from people just like you who all thought they couldn't do this… until they tried it just ONCE. Because once you try it, you'll discover this plan is far easier than you might expect.

Ok, so here's how it works:

On Sunday evening – after my Sunday dinner – I make the conscious decision to take a break from eating. I'll often have a big leisurely Sunday dinner – complete with dessert – at around 7pm. So once the meal is over (around 8pm) I make the decision to take a break from eating.

There is no fanfare or hand-wringing. I make the decision freely and happily. I'm simply "closing the valve" in the same way you'd close the valve to turn off a garden hose.

I'll be sure to drink a little extra water on Sunday evening and when I go to bed I'm fully, happy and my mind is clear.

I wake up Monday morning feeling refreshed and ready to attack the week. While most people are frazzled trying to cram down a quick breakfast while packing a lunch and trying to figure out what to eat for dinner later in the day, I approach my day with a sense of calm and relief.

I won't be eating breakfast today. Instead I enjoy a leisurely cup of coffee with a splash of cream and dash of sugar. Depending on my schedule, I may exercise in the morning. Then shower, drinking plenty more water and arrive at the office ahead of schedule and ready to dive in.

The first few hours of the day are a flurry of activity. My focus and energy levels are sky-high. I get more done during these two initial hours than most people accomplish all day. I sip more water during the morning.

Around 11am, I may feel a slight twinge of hunger. I recognize the sensation and I smile a bit. Because I know that the sensation of hunger will pass shortly. And I know that the slight twinge of hunger means my body is now burning my stored body fat reserves to provide energy.

I have more water – perhaps with a slice of lemon – and dive back into my work. The next two hours pass quickly. I've already accomplished my major objectives for the day. It's 1pm. Time for lunch.

Most of my co-workers will be forced to scarf down a lukewarm burger and fries after picking up dry cleaning and trying to speed through the grocery store to pick everything for dinner.

I enjoy a leisurely hour away from the office. I may go for a walk if the weather is nice. Sometimes I run a few errands or get my car washed. Still other times I'll pop into the local book store and browse the magazines for a while.

I'm free to spend the time however I choose as I'm skipping the practice of eating lunch today.

When I return to the office, I tie up a few loose ends on various projects and prep for a round of meetings. At 2:45pm I start to feel another wave of hunger, but I already know it's coming and I'm ready. I get myself a cup of coffee – black this time—and slowly sip the brew.

By 3pm the coffee is drank, the hunger is gone and I'm wrapped up in a conference call. At this point in the day, others are fighting to keep their eyes open, groggy from lunch. I'm sharp, alert and focused. In a few more hours, I'm done for the day. I pack up my computer, grab another bottle of water for the ride home and I'm on my way.

It's dinner-time when I walk in the door. My wife and kids are happily discussing their day at the dinner table. I set my bags down and pull up a chair. I pour myself a glass of ice cold water. "Daddy you're not eating?" my daughter asks. "Not right now sweetie, I'm not very hungry."

It's not a lie – at this moment I feel zero hunger and I've just imparted the most practical advice on weight loss you can give to a child or an adult: No need to eat if you're not hungry.

We laugh about our day and the next few hours are a blur of homework, bath time and bed time stories. It's nearly 9 pm now, the kids are asleep and I know the next few hours will be the toughest period of the plan.

I'm surrounded by fool… but I'm still choosing to abstain.

It's not always easy – there are a plenty of goodies in the pantry that I'd love to eat. But I drink more water. This time I mix in a special supplement powder that curbs hunger and makes the process easier. (More on this later.) It's now been over 24 hours since I last ate.

Most people NEVER go this long without eating. And it's no coincidence that most people constantly struggle with their weight.

There are a few things around the house that I've been putting off. The light bulb in the bathroom needs to be replaced. A couple bills need to be paid and a load of laundry needs to be folded.

Ordinarily these things would be pushed off "until tomorrow" because dinner and snacking would take precedence. But without the time constraints of a meal, the associated clean-up and the snacking, I have much more free time. I calmly knock out each of the tasks and next thing I know it's 11pm.

I spend the next few minutes talking to my wife about our day, the kids, what's coming up next. Sometimes I find myself exhausted at this point in the day and I'll crawl into bed and quickly fall asleep.

But on this evening, I find myself wide away and with plenty of energy and focus. I don't force anything. I know that my body needs far less sleep during my 44-hour diet.

So I spend a few minutes getting a jump on a work project for the next day. And then I wind down sipping water and tea while watching a documentary I've been meaning to see.

I wake up the next morning feeling somewhat strange. "Hollow" is the only way to describe it. And while it's an odd feeling, it's not uncomfortable. Just different. I also notice I'm feeling warmer than usual.

I know from the research that after 24-32 hours of fasting, your metabolism actually INCREASES so I smile knowing I'm now burning fat at a rapidly accelerated pace.

I don't usually like to exercise during the 2nd day of my fast so my morning is even more leisurely than usual. More water, more coffee. I shower, get the kids off to school and head out to the office.

Along the way, I drink more water mixed with the special supplement powder that cures hunger. Despite that it's been roughly 36 hours since I've eaten, I'm not even hungry.

This sounds shocking to most people, but the research shows that ghrelin levels (the hormone that controls hunger) fall at this point.

I also know that my body is producing growth hormone at 5x higher rates than normal right now and that probably explains why I feel so much younger and energetic at the moment. Plus I noticed a few of the nagging aches and pains we all get past age 35 are dramatically reduced.

Again, the morning is a flurry of focused activity at work and again I've accomplished more in the first few hours than most people accomplish all day. At lunch I pick up a few groceries – knowing that tonight I get to break my fast with a feast.

I'm feeling some moderate levels of hunger now – but the feelings are easy to ignore knowing I'm so close to the finish line. Back to the office for more meetings, more phone calls and more coffee.

Suddenly it's 4pm. It's been roughly 44 hours since I've eaten. I'm not even hungry. I could go even longer but I know there's a point of diminishing returns. I break my fast with an apple and some almonds. T

he nourishment tastes delicious. I be sure to drink more water and then my work day is over and I'm on my way home.

When I get home, the family is at the table. It's taco night! I enjoy a full plate of tacos, beans and rice. And a couple ice-cold "cervezas" for good measure. I feel full and happy. It's only Tuesday but I'm done with my diet for the week.

After dinner, my kids want to go on the trampoline. We bounce around until the sun sets and it's time for bed. Once the kids are in bed, I share a few moments alone with my wife. (Libido is massively increased following re-introduction of food after a fast.)

She drifts to sleep, while I get up and decide to eat again. There's a homemade peach cobbler in the fridge that's been calling my name. I have a 2nd round of tacos, followed by a warm slice of peach cobbler with vanilla ice cream.

In a few minutes I'll be drifting off to sleep. My diet is done for the week. For the rest of the week I can eat all of my favorite foods, enjoy my life without counting calories, calculating macros or weighing anything. I can eat lunch at restaurants with my co-workers, enjoy beer and brats with buddies and cheesecake with my wife.

In the last 44 hours, I've burned more fat than most dieters will burn during an entire week. While others struggle to stick with a diet day in and day out, I can enjoy the rest of my week and not be forced to live my life on a diet.

How To Make The 44 Hour Fast Even Easier

I've been using the 44-hour fast for years now and I've stumbled up some tricks that make the process even easier.

Here are a list of tips and tricks, in no particular order:

Drink plenty of water. This is the single most important key to fasting. If you drink enough water, you will find barely feel any hunger and your energy levels remain stable.

But if you let yourself get dehydrated, you'll suffer through heightened levels of hunger and weakness.

Don't get caught up in scale weight during fasting. If you weigh yourself on day 1 before the fast, you might actually weigh more on day 2 --- despite not eating anything for over 24 hours.

This is simply due to increased water intake. Rest assured, if you fast for 24+ hours you WILL burn fat so even if the scale temporarily goes up due to water weight, you are actually leaner.

Coffee or tea with a small splash of cream or a dash of sugar is fine. If you can handle the taste, black coffee is perhaps nature's finest appetite suppressant.

It's usually better to NOT tell people what you're doing. Most people are nay-sayers and will actively work to sabotage your efforts even if they say they are on your side. There is power in secrecy, so keep your mission to yourself.

Flavored (zero calorie) water or sparkling (zero calorie) water can be a nice change of pace. I will sometimes reward myself with a bottle of sparkling mineral water during the afternoon of my fasts.

Sleep can be strange during your fast. Sometimes I'm exhausted on the first night of my fast and fall asleep as soon as my head hits the pillow. Other times I barely get 2 hrs of sleep.

Try not to worry about it too much. The need for sleep is drastically reduced when fasting. If you can sleep, great. If not, don't stress about it. Enjoy the additional free time.

To that end, I often give myself a reward on the first night of my fast: I'll rent a movie that I've been wanting to see. A guy in my position (busy job, young family) rarely gets a chance to sit down and watch a movie of his own choosing on a Monday night, so this feels like a small luxury to me.

So when I'm going through my day on Monday, I know that come Monday night while the rest of the family sleeps I'll get to enjoy a few hours to myself watching a movie of my own choosing.

I'll often implement a 2nd reward reserved exclusively for Tuesday night (after successfully completing the fast). I'll eat an entire pint of ice cream.

Work to develop fasting amnesia: The first few times you attempt a 44-hour fast, you'll probably find yourself pigging out before the fast... and then again after the fast.

This won't undo the positive effects of a successful 44-hour fast, but it's less than ideal for long-term success.

So work to develop what I call "fasting amnesia." Which means before the fast, don't pig out in advance. Simply eat normal. And after the fast, don't go crazy. Do your best to just eat normally. Eat to fullness – yes. But don't purposefully gorge yourself on junk food or anything like that.

Stay busy. If you have a lot of downtime, you'll find yourself thinking about food a lot and it will make fasting difficult. So do your best to stay busy during your fasts.

I try to schedule haircut appointments or other things that will keep me out of the house as much as possible during my 44 hour fasts because I know the more I'm out of the house the less time there is to be tempted by what's in the pantry.

I like Sunday night to Tuesday afternoon. That's a good schedule for me. I like the regularity of it. But a different 44-hour block may work best for you.

Consider using the 44-hour fast when traveling. One of my clients is a real road warrior and seems to be flying somewhere almost every week. He now uses the 44-hour fast when he travels and loves it.

He says he doesn't have to worry about eating airport food or trying to fight for snacks on the flight. Instead he can just relax, sip a coffee and enjoy the additional free time (not to mention money saved.)

You can workout on your fasting days if you like, but expect performance to suffer. If you can typically bench press 200lbs 10 times, don't be surprised if you can only get 6 or 7 reps when the same workout is performed when fasting.

Don't worry about this: It's a temporary reduction in strength and it will come roaring right back once you resume eating.

At the same time, don't feel that you NEED to exercise during your 44-hour fast. And it goes without saying, if you ever feel light-headed during a workout or at anytime during a fast, SIT DOWN! Drink some additional water and relax. No need to push yourself while fasting.

Abstinence is easier than moderation. Having one bite or one cookie won't automatically ruin your fast, but doing so only makes things harder on yourself.

So do your best to avoid small nibbles or "just a tastes" as those little indiscretions actually make the process more difficult.

It's almost as if the brain ramps up hunger into overdrive when it senses that food is available. And by teasing yourself with little bits, you are sending a message to your brain that food is at the ready.

There is a supplement that can make fasting easier. It's amino acid called "L-Glutamine." You simply mix a teaspoon of the powdered supplement into a glass of water (I prefer zero-calorie flavored water to mask the taste), stir and drink.

Take this supplement 2-3 times per day while fasting and you'll see sharper mental focus and reduced hunger.

Lastly, a warning: You may find the 44-fasting portion of this plan is simply TOO powerful.

Using a weekly 44 hour fast may get you to your goal weight quickly, but continuing to use the 44-hour fast weekly at that point may result in too much weight loss.

In that case, consider using the 44-hour fast only every other week.

Who Should NOT Attempt The 44 Hour Diet?

Here's a quick list of people who should NOT attempt this plan. If you find yourself on this list, don't fret. You can most likely still use the rest of this plan and perhaps in time your situation will change/improve enough to the point where you can us the 44-hour portion of the plan.

Do NOT use the 44-hour diet plan if...

- You are under the age of 18.
- You are currently pregnant or nursing.
- You have a history of fainting or blacking out
- You take medication that must be taken every day and must be taken with food.
- You have a body mass index of less than 18.
- You currently take insulin, metformin or similar drugs.

An Alternative Explanation For Why The 44 Hour Diet Works So Well...

The key to losing weight is creating a caloric deficit. This means consuming fewer calories than it takes to maintain your weight. For example, if you require 2,000 calories to maintain your weight and you only consume 1,900 calories... then your body will tap into your fat stores (remember, fat is just stored energy) to make up the difference.
Most people understand this principle and yet they fail to lose weight because they don't understand that you must create a caloric deficit OVER TIME.

If you need 2,000 calories to maintain your weight, and you only consume 1,900 calories today... but then tomorrow you consume 2,100 calories... well guess what? You won't lose any weight.

To lose weight, you must consume a caloric deficit on a longer time line. By implementing a 44-hour fast at the beginning of the week you are essentially "front-loading" your diet.

You are creating a massive caloric deficit in the beginning of the week. And if you combine a 44 hour fast to kick off the week with a daily target of roughly 1,250 calories over the remainder of the week, rest assumed you will have created a massive caloric deficit over the course of a week.

That's why this plan is actually too powerful for most situations and it's something I only use in the case of extreme circumstances.

The Sinister Reason Why You Haven't Heard About This Plan

I freely admit the idea of using a 44 hour fast once per week to lose weight is certainly not something you hear about every day.   But there's a sinister reason WHY you'll never hear about this approach from the main stream media.

Think about it: A few years ago Subway restaurants were quickly becoming one of the top fast food chains in the world.
But you can only sell so many sandwiches for lunch. So what did they do? Started serving breakfast.

Taco Bell followed suit... and then raised the ante. Not only did Taco Bell start serving breakfast, they doubled-down on their marketing and started pushing the concept of the "4th meal." (a late night meal.)

Make no mistake about it: Getting consumers to eat MORE often is the key to big corporate profits. But they key to getting and staying lean is simple: Eat LESS often. So yes - this diet plan is controversial and probably won't be covered by the mainstream media anytime soon.

And now you know why.

It's Not Just About Looking Good In A Swimsuit...

If you're like most people, you're reading this book because you want to LOOK better – both on the beach and in your street clothes. Ah hell, probably in the bedroom too... right?

There's nothing wrong with that. The 44 Hour Diet can help you get there. But it's not just about looking good. The 44 Hour Diet can drastically improve your health and longevity as well.

In fact, the 44 Hour Diet can actually help you look and feel younger. Here's the proof:

Scientists in Sao Paulo University in Brazil studied the effects of fasting and caloric restriction on groups of rats.

One group of rats ate a normal amount of calories and another group of rats were given 31% less calories.

The group that received the reduced calories actually showed improved collagen density (collagen makes you look younger), thicker cartilage (cartilage makes your joints feel younger) and other signs of reverse aging.

Human studies also show that periods of fasting can not only reverse the signs of aging, but also starve out cancer cells.

Final Thoughts On The 44 Hour Fasting Protocol

"It was so much easier than I thought."

That's the single most common response I get from people attempting a 44-hour fast for the first time.

The idea of a 44-hour fast sounds incredibly difficult. But the reality is that our bodies evolved to go for long periods without food. And an occasional 44-hour fast can not only be health and an incredible tool for losing fat quickly, it's also far easier than most people imagine.

So if you attempt this plan, please drop me a note and let me know how it worked for you. Thank you.

Bonus Chapter: Techniques And Suggestions

Morning Routine

If you do this one thing in the morning, it will take just 60 seconds. But it will help you burn fat all day long.

Here's what this is all about...

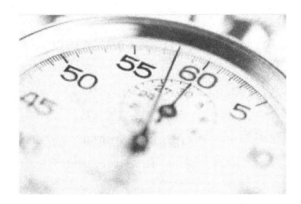

In the 1950's, researchers discovered a hormone in your body called "leptin." Since then it's been studied non-stop as this hormone plays a crucial role in fat burning and leanness.

Leptin is primarily released from fat cells and leptin plays a crucial role in regulating appetite, body fat and metabolism.

How It Works

In simple terms, once released by fat cells leptin travels to the brain where it acts upon leptin receptors inside the hypothalamus in inhibit appetite.

In ever simpler terms: More leptin in your brain makes you eat less.

In theory, if you simply injected leptin into your body it should make you eat less. In fact, scientists tried that with rats and guess what? They took overweight rats, injected them with additional leptin and the rats immediately started eating less, become more active and got thinner.

Success, right? Well, not so fast. In the 1990's they tried this same experiment with overweight humans. But it didn't work! Turns out in overweight human adults, it's not the level of leptin that is the problem, but rather the leptin RECEPTORS in the brain.

In short, if your leptin receptors in your brain are out of balance, increasing leptin won't have the desired effect. And if you're currently carrying excess body fat, there's a good chance your leptin receptors are out of balance.

A Quick Fix?

Researchers were testing sprint training on a group of athletes and found something unusual. Scientist already know that sprint training (exercising as fast and as hard as you can for a very short period of time) can increase heart rate and increase fat burning.

But researchers found that a single 30-second sprint can actually "reset" the leptin receptors in your brain and make you more likely to burn fat for the rest of the day.

Here's The Experiment:

Scientists took a group of adults and had them perform a single "bike sprint" for 30 seconds. This basically means they pedaled as fast as they could for 30 seconds. Then scientist measured leptin levels.

Scientists found that a single 30-second sprint was enough to increase leptin signaling and reset the leptin receptors in your brain.

The 60 Second Morning Routine That Makes You Burn Fat All Day Long

I realize that most people don't have a Wingate bicycle in their bedroom. (A special kind of bike used in the experiment that allows you to adjust the resistance and make it harder to pedal.)

No worries. Here's how to adapt the strategy so you can follow this routine without any equipment.

First, be sure to warm up properly. Some light jogging in place, a few jumping jacks and some easy stretches are just what you need. Rolling out of bed and immediately exercising as hard as you can is recipe for disaster.

Next, perform 60 seconds of either:

- Burpees (if you don't know how to do the exercise, look on the internet "Burpee")
- Mountain-Climbers (if you don't know how to do the exercise, look on the internet "mountain climbers exercise")

Personally, I find burpees way too on the knees so I prefer mountain- climbers but both exercises are good. Both exercises are extremely demanding which is exactly what we want for this routine.

Perform the exercise of your choice for just 60 seconds. Go as fast as you can – safely. You only need to do this for 60 seconds and then you're done. Hooray! You won't burn many calories in just 60 seconds but you'll give your body the signal to reset your leptin receptors which can help boost your metabolism and regular your appetite... all leading to increased fat burning over the rest of the day.

One caveat though: The effects of sprinting on leptin are BLUNTED in the presence of insulin. Translation: For this 60-second routine to work, it needs to be performed on an empty stomach – ideally in the morning when you haven't eaten anything overnight.

So there you have it – the 60 second routine that makes you burn fat all day long.

The Only Ab Exercise You Need

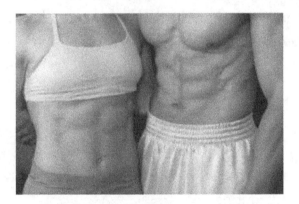

People always think there's a big secret to getting great abs. But guess what? There is NOT. It's really simple. Want great abs? You need to do two things... First, you need to be lean enough to actually SEE your abs. That part comes from diet.

Next, you need to strengthen your abs so they are more visible. That part comes from training.

Training your abs doesn't have to be difficult. In fact, you can great abs with just ONE exercise. Here it is:

The Double Crunch:

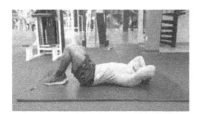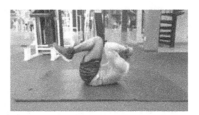

As you can see, with a single movement the double-crunch actually targets both your upper AND lower abs. It's the ultimate "bang for your buck" ab exercise.

Now here's the ultimate "bang-for-your buck" training program. After decades of experience, I've found that abs respond best when you train them nearly every day (5 or 6 days per week) for two weeks, then take two weeks off.

So if I have a beach vacation coming up or some other important event... I'll train my abs every night for 2 weeks straight... and then take the next 2 weeks off and I won't do any ab exercise for the next 2 weeks.

Here's the ultimate training protocol to use with this ab exercise: Do 8 sets of 8 reps. That's 64 total reps.

Start out with 1 minute of rest in between sets. And when that gets too easy, drop down to 45 seconds of rest in between sets. When that gets too easy, drop to 30 seconds of rest between sets.... Then 15 seconds.

When even just 15 seconds of rest between sets gets too easy, then here's how you take things up another level: Start replacing rest time with top position squeezes.

Let me explain:

Let's say you've done your first set of 8 reps. Instead of resting for 15 seconds, hold the top position (where your knees are touching your elbows) and squeeze/tighten/flex your abs as hard as you can.

Do this for 5 seconds to start. And then once you can do a 5 second squeeze between all sets, gradually start to INCREASE the time.

So there you have it – the only ab exercise you need to get great abs.

The Emergency Transformation Plan

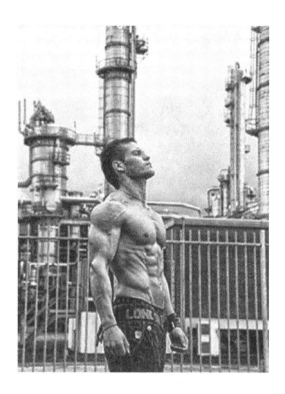

I get a lot of emails that sound something like this:

"Help!! I'm going on vacation in two weeks and I want to get ripped and muscular so I can finally look good on the beach! Can you help me????"

For some reason people always use a bunch of punctuation marks when desperate.

The truth is, I actually CAN help. Don't get me wrong. I'm not saying I can make you look like a professional bodybuilder in 9 days.

But I CAN help you slash fat, add lean mass and reshape your physique in just 9 days. It won't be easy, but here's the plan:

Step #1: 20 Hours Of Fasting Per Day

To maximize fat loss, we need to give your body the maximum amount of time to burn fat.

When does your body burn stored body fat? Well, to make a complicated subject simple, your body burns the most fat when your stomach is empty.

So for that reason, we are going to spend approximately 20 hours a day in a "fasted" (or unfed) state.

That leaves a 4 hour window for eating. Typically people will end up eating either one massive meal in that two hour window or 2-3 medium sized meals. So that answers the question of "when to eat" but how about "what to eat".

Step #2: Eat This

There are only a couple rules here. The first is that you will NOT consume any liquid calories. That's right, no protein shakes, no alcohol, no juice or soda.

Diet drinks, coffee, tea are all ok, but water is far and away the single best choice during these 9 days.

Next, we're going to focus on protein. You are going to SHOOT for 1 gram of protein per pound of bodyweight. So if you weigh 200lbs, that's 200 grams of protein per day.

If you want to have MORE, that's ok. And there will be some days where you just can't eat enough protein. That's ok too.

The key is to make getting your daily protein the CORNERSTONE of your meals. This will force you to choose better foods and force you to consume beef, chicken, fish, eggs instead of opting for junk foods.

You are certainly allowed to consume fats and carbohydrates on this plan but the focus is on protein.

Step #3: 500 Daily Reps

So now we're creating a massive caloric deficit via our eating strategy. This will force our body to start burning away body fat.

But we can speed up the process a bit more and signal the body to retain muscle AND even pack on new muscle. The key: 500 daily reps.

By making 500 daily reps of a given exercise your goal, you will be forced to get up out of your chair and move around. This will speed up fat loss. But you will also be shocking your body and providing a new catalyst for growth.
I recommend one of the following options for your daily 500 reps: Push-ups
Sit-ups Bodyweight Squats Kettlebell Swings Dumbbell/Barbell Curls (if you have access to a light set of weights)

Pick an exercise and knock out 500 reps over the course of the day. You are NOT trying to get all 500 reps in one shot. You are not trying to go to failure.

You are simply doing reps throughout the day in the attempt to accumulate 500 total reps.

So you might do 50 push ups right up waking up, another 50 before you get in the shower. 2 sets of 25 after your morning coffee, and so on and on until you've racked up 500 total reps.

You can vary the exercise selections throughout the nine days but no in a given day. In other words, do NOT do 100 sit ups, 100 pushups, 100 squats, 100 swings and 100 curls in a day. But it is OK to do 500 pushups one day, then 500 swings the next day, then 500 bodyweight squats the next day, etc.

Step #4: The 60/20 Workout

This is my favorite routine to use when I need to get results in a hurry. The concept is simple: You load up a barbell with a given weight and then attempt to get 60 reps in 20 minutes.

If you are able to train 5 days a week, then you will simply perform one 20 minute workout per training day.

If you are only able to train 2 or 3x a week, then you will perform two 20 minute blocks per training session.

Here are some of my favorite ways to use this routine: If you are able to train 5x a week (Mon – Friday): Monday: 60/20 Barbell Squats
Tuesday: 60/20 Close Grip Bench Press Wednesday: 60/20 Power Cleans
Thursday: 60/20 Close Grip Weighted Chins Friday: 60/20 Deadlifts

So let's use Monday as an example. You first do a general warm-up and then head to the squat rack.

Warm up with some lighter weights and then move to your working weight. Typically you will want to select a weight that would allow you to get between 7-10 reps if you trying to get as many reps as possible in one set.

Let's say you are good for 10 reps with 315lbs so you decide to use 315lbs. You will set a timer (or just check the clock) for 20 minutes and then it's your goal to get 60 reps.

You can break up the reps any way you want. Most often people will knock out around 10 reps with their first set, take a quick break, try and get a few sets of 7, a few sets of 5, and by the end you'll be grinding out singles.

Because we are dealing with a tight timeline, it is actually better to be too aggressive rather than too conservative. If you are actually able to complete all 60 reps in 20 minutes, you went too light.

But if you are only able to do 30 reps in 20 minutes you went too heavy. The sweet spot is a weight that allows you to get somewhere around 45 – 55 reps in 20 minutes.

Again, you are TRYING to get 60 but it is better to bust your ass and only get 55 rather than getting all 60 and realizing you went way too light. If you get all 60 reps, plan to increase the weight next time.

If you didn't get all 60 reps, keep the weight the same next time you perform this exercise and attempt to get more reps.

Split for someone training 3x per week:

Monday: Barbell Squats & CG Bench Press (60/20 for each, so essentially a 40 minute workout.)

Wednesday: CG Weighed Chins& Deadlifts Friday: Power Cleans & Weighted Dips ########

Those are my two favorite splits. Obviously they are barbell-based as that's what I feel is most effective given only 9 days to get somebody into better shape.

But if barbells are not an option for you due to circumstances of injury, you can easily swap out dumbbells or machine variations.

Just try to focus on compound exercises and stick with the rule of shooting for 60 reps in 20 minutes.

A Word About Supplements

I'm not a big fan of supplements and most times I don't take anything at all in regards to supplements. But again, if we're talking about making a massive change in just 9 days it might make sense to take the following supplements.

#1) Creatine Monohydrate: Take 10 grams per day (5 grams in the a.m., 5 grams in the p.m) during the course of the 10 days as this can help with strength, muscle mass and muscle fullness.

I have no specific product recommendations. Just get your basic Creatine Monohydrate powder. Don't fall for any of the marketing hype.

The cheap, basic stuff works just fine and the more expensive "bells and whistles" in the other versions don't do anything but inflate the price tag.

#2) A Fat-Burner: I don't believe that any fat burning pill will actually help you burn fat, but they can help suppress your appetite and if this is your first time going 20 hours a day fasted, you might appreciate the help.

Again, I don't have any specific product recommendations as I don't take any fat burning supplements (black coffee works just fine) but if you want some help with appetite control this might be something to look in to.)

Q&A

#1) Does it matter what time I train do the 60/20 workouts?

A: The best situation is if you can do the 60/20 workout right at the end of your 20 hour fast so you can immediately start eating.

If that works for you, great. Do that. But otherwise it doesn't matter. If you have to do the 60/20 workout at 7am and then you don't eat until 8pm at night, then that's just what you have to do.

#2) Shouldn't I eat something after my workout? Shouldn't I at least drink a protein shake?

A: If you can line it up so your workout is right before your eating window, then great. But otherwise you will NOT eat anything after your workout. It's only for 9-10 days, you can handle it.

#3) This just seems like a LOT... I'm worried about overtraining.

A: It is a lot. Because to make an impressive transformation in just 9 days you've got to push the pedal to the floor. And yes, you WILL be overtrained during this block of time. This is intentional. We are going to push you hard for 9 days to get you in top shape. Assuming you are using this plan to get in shape for a beach vacation, you will have EARNED the right to sit on the beach for a week and eat as much food as you want.

Your body will recover during this time and instead of getting fat and out of shape on your vacation you will be getting recovered and rested up. When you get back to "real life" you will be rested and ready to jump right in to a saner, long-term training and diet plan.

#4) Can I use this strategy for more than 9 days?

A) You could conceivablly use this strategy for 10-14 days max but I wouldn't push it any more than that.

How To Kill Fat Cells And Avoid Rebound Weight Gain

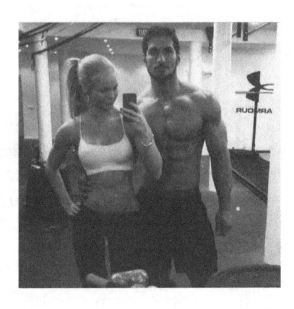

Here's some unfortunate science for you:

When you overeat, your body stores fat.

I'm sure this much you already know. But did you know how YOUR body stores fat?

Well, it's very simple. At first your body will just store the extra fat inside your existing fat cells.

But when those existing fat cells can no longer hold all the extra fat, your body starts to create NEW fat cells.

When you lose fat, your fat cells will release their fat contents into the blood stream. In other words, you fat cells will shrink.

But... the number of fat cells you have doesn't change! Fat cells don't die, they just hang around waiting for you to get fat again. And guess what, research shows that the more fat cells you have, the more hunger you experience so it's only a matter of time until you do in fact get fat again.

Unless...

You KILL These Extra Fat Cells!

Until very recently, it was thought to be impossible to kill fat cells. But we now know there are a few different strategies you can use to kill fat cells. Here they are...

Cold Exposure: Research has shown that exposing fat to cold actually speeds the death of fat cells. A cold shower is a great start (good for testosterone levels too) but for the full effect you want to try an ice bath where you keep your body submerged in ice or cold water for 20-30 minutes.

(Obviously, you need to use caution here. Ice baths require proper medical supervision.)

Sunlight and Vitamin D supplementation: Sunlight has also been shown to kill fat cells. That may be one reason why you seem to lose fat when you go on a tropical vacation. Try supplementing with 3,000 – 5,000 I.U.s of liquid Vitamin D3 to speed the killing of fat cells.

High Intensity Exercise: While we know that losing fat only shrinks fat cells, it appears that high-intensity exercise actually speeds up the death of fat cells. This may be one reason why sprinting-based fat loss program are so effective.

Try to find a way to work a sprinting type conditioning program into your weekly workouts – even just one day a week – and you'll be speeding the death of your empty fat cells.

Eat berries every day. Berries – specifically blueberries, raspberries, blackberries and strawberries contain something called polyphenols which have been shown to speed fat cell death.

Shoot for 2-3 cups of berries almost daily to accelerate death of fat cells.

A German research study showed that consuming 3-6 grams of CLA (Conjugated Linoleic Acid) can kill fat cells.

Remember, the best way to LOSE fat is still with an aggressive caloric deficit but once you've lost the fat try these fat-cell killing techniques to help you stay lean for life.

CPSIA information can be obtained
at www.ICGtesting.com
Printed in the USA
LVHW051946221220
674884LV00006B/164

9 781801 443159